The New Rules Of Weight Loss

Richard Clarke

TABLE OF CONTENTS

INTRODUCTION

Today's world is suffering from the effects of bad food, bad water and most of all bad and confusing advice. This book will help you to cut through the confusion and give you a clear idea of how to improve your health, fitness and energy.

Over the last 18 years I have witnessed many of the "old" rules being replaced by "new" rules which, sometimes, were the exact opposite of what we previously believed.

The governments and food manufacturers of this world, together tend to set the health agendas and the ultimate advice that is given out to the masses.

The information and advice given by governments is often "evidence based", which sounds great but in reality the research has more holes in it than a string vest, is dated, and by the time it's published and reaches "the people on the street" is out of touch with what is working.

I worked for the government in Wales for over 10 years in the areas of health and fitness and I saw first hand that the information being given was not helping the majority of people.

Due to the limitations placed upon most people's time, I will aim to make this book a concise summary of what I see as the New Rules Of Weight Loss.

In fourteen short chapters I will reveal the major changes that I have seen happen during my career so far, and outline what the "RULES OF WEIGHT LOSS" actually are right now.

CHAPTER ONE

The Wrong End Of The Stick? The main goal should be...

Old Rule: The main goal of your diet and exercise should be WEIGHT LOSS

New Rule: The main goal of your diet and exercise plan should be HEALTH

Top Tip: when we talk about weight loss we usually mean fat loss. For the purposes of this book I will use the terms fat loss and weight loss interchangably

Let me explain my feathered friend... as a younger man, just like nowadays, I was employed to help people set and achieve their goals.

Looking back I probably had one of the hardest client groups - people sent for exercise by their GP. They were very unwell people, took multiple forms of medication, and lived in the 3rd most deprived area of Wales(UK), Llanelli.

The most common reasons for referral would be being overweight and depressed. So we would sit down in my little office and draw out all these different targets and then set

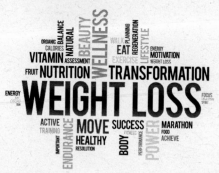

about achieving them.

Weight loss would usually be the MAIN goal. We would chase the weight loss at all costs because that is what they (thought) they wanted.

The scheme was good, but the weight loss results were variable at best.

Train hard and diet hard (the dieticians usually set the diets).

Lose a bit of weight.
Repeat the process.
Maybe lose some more weight.

Then at some point they would stop losing weight.

So we would then do the "logical" thing and train a bit harder, if that was even an option for some, and cut back on the food some more.

But still there would be no weight loss, they were stuck, some even gained weight back.

So this went on for years. Very mixed results to be honest.

I have subsequently learned where I was going wrong.

The main goal, for a diet, fitness and WEIGHT loss plan should

be to get healthier NOT LOSE WEIGHT.
Good health leads to weight loss, not the other way around.

Chasing weight loss can actually make you unhealthy.

Let me tell you a little story. I was having a chat with a lady in the gym the other day. She was "starting back" (again).

"How's the training going?" I asked her.

"It's ok at the minute, but ask me again in a couple of weeks." She said.

"Why, what do you mean?"

"Every time I try to get fit and lose some weight I do really well for a few weeks and then I usually get ill."

This is something that is very common, so I thought I would share some practical advice to make your life a bit easier when you decide to do some good clean eating and some quality training.

Here is the scenario: you are all "ready and motivated" to go on a stint of healthy eating and exercise. You do well for a few weeks, even a month or more, and then you get ill.

You take a week or two off, sometimes longer and before you know it you have to start from scratch again.

I expect this sounds familiar and you want to know why it happens.

Firstly, and most importantly, I would never criticise someone who has made the EFFORT to stick to a regime for any period of time. It shows a desire to change and you cannot do much without that. But those EFFORTS need to be directed elsewhere.

Getting fit and healthy is not as straightforward as most people think. Otherwise more people would be in shape right?

You have to do things in the right order to get long lasting success. You need to point your enthusiasm in the right direction.

Just like when you build a house: if you get the order of events wrong then you are going to get into trouble further down the line.

If you are not healthy enough strict dieting and intense exercise will make you ill. You have to reclaim your health first (via sleep, reducing stress, not drinking like a fish and eating better). Then get fit after that.

People naturally associate losing weight with exercise and dieting, and they combine the two together for maximum results. That is kind of right but not right if you are a beginner.

Diet and exercise combined just burns you out and puts extra stress on your body. Exercise stresses the body and puts your immune system under pressure. That is the reason the lady gets ill every time she goes on a diet and exercises.

Her immune system cannot take it just yet. She "runs herself down" by restricting her food and doing the exercise. She should just start a bit slower and should not try to do it all in the first month.

She should stick to healthy eating at first and just walking.

The message is to make sure you do not go like a bull at a gate and chase WEIGHT LOSS at the cost of your HEALTH.

Take the energy and enthusiasm you have to do exercise and put it into learning how to make some clean and tasty recipes, like the ones from my cookbooks (www.richard-

clarke.co.uk).
If you are serious about change and are in it for the long haul it is always worth taking some time to get healthier first.

So if getting healthier is the key, what things cause us to become unhealthy in the first place?

Most people in the Western World die from diseases of excess. So obviously at this point it would be easy to say environment and lifestyle factors cause us to become unhealthy, sick and ultimately die, which is true.

The things that cause us to go down the wrong route and GAIN WEIGHT are the bad habits we expose ourselves to on a daily basis - the environment and lifestyle influences really mess up the insides of our bodies, our health and our FAT LOSS.

What you need to avoid:

- Acidity – it's better to have an alkaline body as opposed to an acidic one if you want to be healthy, disease resistant and able to LOSE FAT more easily (more in chapter 7).

- Inflammation – controlling inflammation means controlling health, disease and FAT LOSS (more in Chapter 8)

- Deficiency – balancing deficiencies is key to avoiding sickness, disease and maximizing FAT LOSS (more in chapter 12)

- Disease – avoiding disease as far as possible and looking after your immune system will promote best health and FAT LOSS

I will discuss each of these subjects in turn throughout the book.

CHAPTER TWO

THEY TOLD ME A CALORIE WAS JUST A CALORIE

Old Rule: A calorie is just a calorie

**New Rule: All calories are not created equal.
The makeup of each calorie is more important than the calorific value itself.**

Ok this one was rammed down my neck as an undergraduate.

"A calorie is a calorie is a calorie", they said. A calorie is a measure of energy.

When people talk about calories they usually refer to Kcal (kilocalories).

Technically one Kcal is the energy required to heat 1 gram of water by 1 degree C.

Carbohydrates and proteins contain around 4-5Kcal per gram and fats contain 9Kcal per gram.

Knowing all this, we then were encouraged to work out

people's energy balance and come up with programmes to burn 3500 Calories (or one pound of fat) or more per week.

To calculate someone's energy balance you need to know how many calories he or she burned (-) compared to how many calories they consumed (+).

It would leave you with an amount of calories - usually people were eating MORE calories than they burned, that's why they had gained weight.

Then we would switch it around so they were consuming LESS calories than they were burning to create a DEFICIT, and hey presto – weight loss would follow, kinda.

The thing is it didn't work for everyone and it didn't work all of the time.

The trouble was, following this theory people were allowed to eat whatever the hell they wanted, as long as it was within their calorific allowance.

They avoided high calorie foods such as butter and nuts in favour of things like pasta, cereal and fruit. That's just madness.

Some people tested the "calorie is a calorie theory" to the max and ate EMPTY CALORIE foods such as Mars bars, bread and so on and never lost any weight DESPITE being in deficit/negative energy balance.

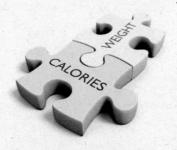

So overtime the calorific model became useless, well nearly.

These days we know that the content of each meal is FAR more important than its calorific value - hence the change in rules from "a calorie is just a calorie" to "all calories are not created equal".

You can consume a diet with higher calories containing more of the RIGHT foods and lose weight. And the opposite is true - you can consume a lower calorie diet of poor foods, and STILL GAIN weight.

The reality of the matter is most people CAN'T over consume foods that are healthy.

Many people have shunned NUTS due to their high calorific value, but it's been proven that when someone adds nuts to their diet they don't usually gain weight.

In fact some studies have proven that nuts may actually help weight control, which may be due to their effect on appetite. *(García-Lorda P, et al. Nut consumption, body weight and insulin resistance. European Journal of Clinical Nutrition. 2003;57 Suppl 1:S8-11)*

The reason is that your body uses food for two main purposes:

1. Fuel
2. Building materials

The fact the body needs building materials for making hormones, bone, blood muscle and so on is what the OLD RULE did not consider.

Your body will respond better to good food calories from building materials, than just any old JUNK calories.

So if your body is going to be healthy, we need to nourish it with high-density nutrition foods, regardless of calories to a point.

The calorie model fails to take into account lots of other variables that we know affect weight loss such as appetite and hormonal control (more on that in chapter 12).

CHAPTER THREE

Carbs, Low Carbs or No Carbs? (Carbohydrates – part 1)

Old Rule: Eat 6-11 portions a day (government food pyramid)

New Rule: Carbohydrates need to be monitored and are activity dependent

This is a biggie, hence the two parts.

First off let's just be clear when we say carbohydrates what we mean. There are two types of carbohydrates, complex and simple.

The complex ones are referred to as just carbs or starches and the simple carbohydrates referred to as sugars.

Carbohydrates are a big issue and they cause huge problems (soooo many people are carbohydrate addicts).

I'm *not* a fan of no carbs unless it's done in a structured way, but I *am* very much for the low carb approach.

Low carbs, depending on how big you are, is about 100g or less a day. That equates to:

- a standard (150g) portion of blue berries contains 20g of sugar
- a large apple contains 23g of sugar
- a large portion (200g) of broccoli contains 14g of sugar
- a large (200g) portion of spinach contains 7g of sugar
- a small (150g) baked potato contains 30g of sugar

Total = 96g of sugar

Notice how much higher the fruit is in sugar than vegetables - also vegetables contain comparable amounts of protein per gram.

Top Tip: Load up of green veggies and keep fruit to 1-2 portions a day to boost health, vitality and of course WEIGHT LOSS

People call LOW CARB different things, but it's essentially the same:
- Paleo
- High Protein
- Low Carb

I often call it "Healthy Atkins".

Call it what you will the plan looks a bit like this.

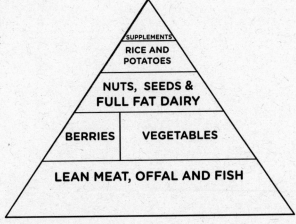

Let's start with saying which foods are classed as carbohydrates:

- Bread, rice, pasta, potatoes.
- Fruit
- Vegetables
- Honey
- Alcohol
- Fizzy drinks

Since 1992 the government and its army of dieticians has been responsible for advising people to follow the food pyramid, and more recently, the food plate guidelines, regarding your nutritional intake.

They have obviously made a big cock up because the country has never been so fat and unhealthy.

These guidelines currently suggest that about 33% of your food intake should be in the form of carbohydrates such as bread, rice, potatoes and pasta, and another 33% to come from fruit and vegetables. The situation is even worse for diabetics, which I will explain later in this chapter.

So why are carbohydrates so bad?

Where do I start...

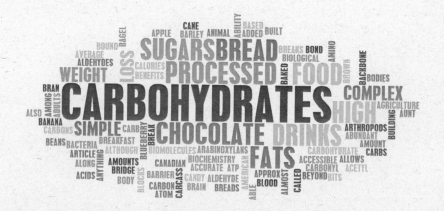

Carbs, No carbs or Low Carbs?

Two of the main problems with many carbohydrates are that they:

1. Provide little or no nourishment in the form of vitamins and minerals
2. They increase the hormone INSULIN and thus fat storage

(Before anyone asks, you don't need starchy carbs for FIBER, you can get better sources of fiber from vegetables and nuts.)

Let me share a story about the time I went to a restaurant for a birthday party:

It was my niece's 6th birthday party, everyone was there. We were all placing our orders and I noticed that on the menu there was the option for "bottomless" drinks and unlimited fries.

Now I have worked in America in my younger days and I knew exactly what this is, in case you don't already know it basically means "all you can eat and drink" of the fizzy drinks and fries.

Let me tell you now that my family ordered at least THREE extra bowls of fries and someone at the table had THREE pints of coke.

Three pints of coke! That's 39 spoons of sugar. (Could you eat 39 tea spoons of sugar?)

One of the main reasons people put on weight is basically because of things like bread, biscuits, alcohol, sugar in all its forms (from fruit to sweets and chocolate).
It's like this:

1. When you drink 1.5 litres of coke (or consume lots of carbohydrates or ANY large meal for that matter) you will have a MASSIVE rise in blood sugar and subsequently a MASSIVE release of insulin.

2. Insulin is a GROWTH and massive FAT STORAGE hormone, and if it's in your system you can't lose weight effectively.

NOTE: Carbohydrates and insulin are like the first two dominoes, when they fall they knock lots of other dominoes over, which also affect your health and weight gain such as – hormones, appetite, stress, toxins and your environment

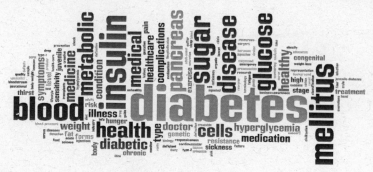

(which we will cover in the book).

What Types & When Should You Eat Them?

The best types of starchy carbohydrates are rice and potatoes. From personal experience I prefer basmati or brown rice and either normal or sweet potatoes.

You should eat your starchy carbohydrates within an hour AFTER exercise or activity as a general rule. It's called BACK LOADING.

You should BACK LOAD with carbohydrates and eat them once you have first depleted your stores.

With simple carbohydrates like berries, they can be best eaten for breakfast (also a time when your stores are depleted).

If you do not exercise (or on non-exercise days), for best

WEIGHT LOSS, you will probably be able to get along just fine on some meat, good fats, and some berries and vegetables.

When did fruit become bad?

Fruit is meant to be healthy right?
5 a day and all that. Well, yes and no...

Let me tell you what has changed.

Yes – fruit is still full of great natural sugars and vitamins and in essence is still healthy.

But (and a big BUT) it's NOT so good for those looking to lose weight when eaten IN LARGE QUANTITIES. On the blog I told the story about a client of mine having fruit smoothies for breakfast "because they're healthy". Trouble was he wasn't losing any weight.

So I checked his food diary and he was having about 9-10 portions of fruit per smoothie each day.

That's just simply too much sugar, fruit or not.

Yes the sugar in fruit is natural fructose, but that's still too much for the body TO LOSE WEIGHT (it all relates back to the release of too much insulin).

If you are trying to lose weight, I generally recommend eating NO MORE THAN 1-2 portions of berries or fruit a day (plus loads of GREEN veggies).

If you are NOT trying to lose weight, put this book down and crack on with your 5 a day or whatever you are doing.

The next question I invariably get asked is "which fruit is BEST to eat to lose weight?".

This is the boring, yet important sciencey bit.

The answer is LOW G.I. fruit. (also known as – low carb fruit). G.I. means glyceamic index, which basically indicates how much sugar is in the food. Every food/fruit has a score on the glyceamic index. The GI of a food ranges from 1-100, high meaning more sugar low GI meaning less sugar.

Science lecture over. What you really want to know is this...

The 5 Best Low Carb Fruits (eat these more frequently)

1. Berries (blueberries, raspberries)
2. Cherries
3. Plums
4. Grapefruits
5. Apples

5 Worst High Carb Fruits (eat these less frequently)

1. Watermelon/Cantaloupe (honeydews are the ok ones)
2. Banana
3. Pineapple
4. Grapes
5. Mango

This is not a definitive list, there are plenty of other high and low carb fruits, just google "GI food list".

CHAPTER FOUR

Carbohydrates & Diabetes (Carbohydrates - part 2)

Old Rule: Diabetics should follow a HIGH carbohydrate and low fat diet

New Rule: Diabetics should follow a LOW carbohydrate diet with a moderate fat intake

To be perfectly honest I never thought I would be talking about some of the things in this book never mind this chapter.

It's a controversial discussion and I will be explaining to you why many people including some of my clients are going completely against government nutrition guidelines and their doctor's advice when it comes to diabetes

Sound crazy? Read on my friend and maybe you will learn something completely new about diabetes, especially if you are a diabetic struggling to lose weight.

Diabetes is a generic term used when a person's blood sugar is above normal levels. This rise in blood sugar is caused either by the pancreas not providing enough insulin or due to the cells not responding to the insulin produced (called insulin resistance).

Top Tip: Exercising improves insulin sensitivity and reduces insulin resistance.

About 3.8 million people in the UK have diabetes, but the charity Diabetes U.K. have made predictions that that could become high as 6.2 million by 2035/2036.

These figures do not include the many people who often go undiagnosed. It's been suggested that including these undiagnosed people would treble the total figure. It's a can of worms the NHS doesn't want to open, as the implications could be huge.

Silent Killer

There are not many symptoms of having diabetes and people are often "picked up" as having it whilst having general checkups or treatment for other things. That's the silent bit.

It just creeps up on you and you can't see it coming.

Symptoms which are so mild they are easy to miss, and even easier to ignore. The easiest way to check if you are at risk is getting your blood sugars tested. It can be done for free by the nurse at the surgery.

You can also do it at home, but you will need a glucose meter or a self-test kit. I have seen self tests for £5 on amazon, which have all the instructions and are easy to use.

The reading will tell you two things, what your "fasted" blood sugar actually is and if it's normal or there is any reason to

see a GP. A GP will usually do at least two more tests to confirm that you have either pre-diabetes or diabetes.
There are three main types of diabetes, type 1, type 2 and the third is called gestational diabetes (during pregnancy).

This chapter is mostly related to people who suffer from type 2 diabetes or DIET controlled diabetes as it is often called.

People who suffer from type 2 diabetes do so because their cells fail to respond and use insulin properly, known as insulin resistance.

Type 2 diabetes is the most common form and around 90% of diabetes sufferers in the UK have type two diabetes. Obese people often suffer from type 2.

We are told by GP's, health practitioners, government dieticians and many other people 'in the know', not to do certain things, so we listen and do what they say.

When I worked with GP referrals for 6 years, the recommendations that we used to see, given by the dieticians, to diabetics, were incorrect, but I did not know this at the time.

Now, if you are a diabetic, and have been given (and followed) this advice (high carb low fat), you would have more than likely gained weight, the opposite of your goal I would guess.

I'm not saying doctors recommend the wrong thing on purpose (they do what they are trained to do).

It would be a risk for a doctor to recommend to their patient to do something that goes against the normal grain, doctors back up all of the theories by saying it is 'evidence based' whereas in reality there is often a lot of evidence that also proves its ineffectiveness. However, at the very least I would think the doctors, and people who are there to help diabetics, need to take a second look at this area, and fast.

It's a messed up situation.

I would also say that you should never make any changes without first discussing things with your doctor or diabetic nurse.

So what are type 2 diabetes sufferers being told by their doctors?

They are being told that the best way to treat their condition is to follow a diet high in carbohydrates and low in fat. On the NHS website it recommends that people who suffer from type 2 diabetes consume starchy carbohydrates with each meal!

What is wrong with this? You should have an idea already but... it's the INSULIN again.

The diabetics and pre diabetics already have reduced sensitivity to the hormone, and their bodies are totally drowning in the stuff.

In recent years, there is an increasing movement that suggests that following a low carb diet is better for type 2 diabetes sufferers.

There are very few doctors who recommend this, as it goes away from what they have been trained.

Diabetes is a condition that responds better to nutritional improvements than it does medication.

The advice given by GPs, dieticians and groups like Diabetes UK is misleading for diabetics. The information is making it harder for them to control their blood sugar and is unnecessarily putting them at a higher risk of other complications.

Did You Know?

Before modern medicine, back in the old days, before insulin injections were discovered, diabetes was treated with

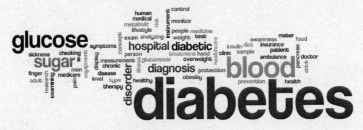

a...(drum roll)... low carb diet.

The doctors back then, who were true masters of their trade if you ask me, took a logical view that if diabetics couldn't control their blood sugar levels, then they should not eat any sugar or starchy carbohydrates.

It makes sense.

However.... "Common sense is not always common practice"

They replaced that logical approach with the one we currently have. More and more diabetics are discovering the massive benefits that low carb eating can have on their health.

Dr Spence, a regular contributor to the British Medical Journal (BMJ), questions the conventional wisdom of doctors who recommend various different medications to lower blood sugar levels, when there is no evidence that this leads to health benefits such as reduced risk of heart disease or death. From what I have found, a diet made up of quality eggs, fish, meat, nuts, seeds, good oils, some fruits and plenty of green leafy vegetables, is the best way to control blood sugar levels and reduce the negative effects associated with type 2 diabetes.

Diabetics can't handle sugar so why are they being advised to eat a diet rich in sugar? It doesn't make sense.

Can We Trust Them?

My Dad calls them lying bastards (LB) and I think he is not far off. The LBs in question are PURPOSELY giving out misleading information.

I want to share a few examples of the DECEIT and LIES being told by our own government and Diabetes UK.

See the thing is, organisations like diabetes UK and NHS recommend a diet that is totally unsuitable for diabetics.

They recommend up to 14 portions of starchy carbs a day which for non-diabetics is too much, but for a diabetic it's just crazy.

They seem totally unwilling to admit there is any problem with the overconsumption of carbohydrate based foods. It seems, to me at least, that the NHS and Diabetes UK are always coming down on the wrong side of the argument.

I think we should all have a healthy cynicism toward the government and organisations like diabetes UK, and we certainly shouldn't believe everything they tell us.

It seems that for now, you can't rely on them to give impartial advice that allows us to be healthy.

Why would they do this? I'm not sure really... but...

- Maybe because saying carbs are "bad" would have legal implications.
- If everyone goes on a low carb diet, businesses and the food chain will be affected.
- They can prescribe more drugs and medication if people are unhealthy.

Make of it what you want and make your own mind up. I know what I think, LB

Resource www.diabetes.co.uk. NOT to be confused with Diabetes UK.

This forum thread in particular is interesting - diabetics are talking about what they are told to do and what they actually do.

http://www.diabetes.co.uk/forum/threads/carbs-or-not.39928/

CHAPTER FIVE

Fat - They Pick On Me Just Because I'm Fat

Old Rule: Low fat is GOOD. Fat, especially saturated fat is BAD for you and causes heart disease and high cholesterol.

New Rule: Low fat is BAD. Fat, especially saturated fats, are essential for the body, are good for your heart and do not directly affect cholesterol. (see cholesterol chapter)

Fat doesn't make you fat.

Ok so we now know from the last chapter that amongst other things, it's the starchy carbs and sugar that make most people gain weight.

But for a very long time many people believed that the best way to lose BODY fat was simply by cutting out fats from their diets, specifically saturated fat.

Over the years many of us have been bombarded by of visions of the saturated fat in their food clogging up their arteries.

Most diet enthusiasts or people trying to eat healthily will look at the back of a packet see a high fat content and put it straight back on the shelf. I have heard people say "as long as its 3% fat or less I can have it". Fat has become demonised.

The "low fat" crew become blind to the fact that we need fats in our diet and were only concerned in avoiding anything high in fat, especially the saturated kind.

Big mistake.

Why do we need fats?

Your brain is over 60% fat.

The fat you eat gets turned into the building materials for your hormones, especially saturated fat. If you want to feel good it's pretty important to eat fat. Fats make up a crucial part of a well balanced diet, a well balanced diet will help you with fat loss, and so eating fat can help you lose fat.

Fats are necessary for energy, if you cut out all of your fats you would feel tired and fatigued and be unable to do anything properly.

Fat helps to boost your immune system, aids brain functioning, stops harmful diseases and without it your hair, skin, nails and joints would suffer.

Eating fats is a great way of filling you up and helps to prevent you from snacking on junk foods, as well as that, fats are rich in flavour!

Low Fat Diets

A low fat diet will make you feel like rubbish and throw your hormones out of balance and often leads to depression.

If you see low fat, it means HIGH SUGAR. The fat has been removed and replaced with sugar. There is a massive problem.

After many years we now know that LOW FAT DIETS make people gain weight.

There are many low in fat substitutes which I will tell you to stay well clear of, things like low fat crisps yoghurts and cereal bars.

In my opinion people need to be eating MORE fat and less carbohydrates.

It is important though that it is the right type of fats.

Bad Fats and Good Fats

There are still good fats and bad fats.

The bad ones these days would be too much omega 6 (vegetable oils) and trans-fats.

Cooking, at high temperatures such as frying, and deep frying, with vegetable oil and olive oils and alike, is not recommended as the fats are not able to withstand those temperatures, and lose their benefits and become inflammatory.

The good fats you need to be consuming include nuts, seeds, extra virgin olive oil, coconut oil, butter, meat, eggs, avocados and fish.

Coconut oil is a good product to buy, you should use it for cooking and it supplies a good source of omega 3 fatty acids that are anti-inflammatory.

Coconut milk is also another good ingredient you should try.

If you struggle to include fish in your diet I would recommend purchasing a good quality fish oil supplement.

You should also eat good quality eggs and red meat, as there are lots of hormones boosting fats in there.

The fat found in red meat and eggs can boost a man's testosterone significantly.

You should swap margarine for normal organic butter

It is still true if you ate a diet high in fatty foods such as chips, burgers, pastries, pizza and fried chicken, you would be more prone to gain weight.

There are four different types of fats. All of which have specific functions and affect our body in a different way:

1. Saturated fats - You get saturated fats from foods such as meat, eggs, butter, dairy and products such as coconut oil.

2. Monounsaturated fats - You will find these mostly in foods such as avocados, peanuts and olive oil.

3. Polyunsaturated fats - These fats give you the essential fatty acids we need, omega 3 and omega 6. The best sources of omega 3 fatty acids come from oily fish and grass fed meat. For omega 6 - meat, eggs and seeds are the best sources.

4. Trans fats - Last but not least is trans fats. Trans fats do naturally   occur in small quantities, but most of the time trans fats are artificially created. You will find the highest source of trans fats come from cheap processed foods.

Feed Your Brain FATS

In the future, more people will die from mental health than

from cardiovascular disease, one of the bi-products of living longer lives, our brains wear out before our hearts and lungs.

I will give you some pointers to help keep your brain healthy.

Top Tip: There is a level of saturated fat contained in every type of fatty food, it's been argued, why would nature create a food containing something which is trying to make you healthier alongside something which is trying to kill you? It doesn't really make sense!

I believe all natural fats are good for us in the right amounts, including saturated fat.

The truth is we can't live very well without fat, low fat diets proved that.

Our cell membranes are made up mostly from fat (70%), considering we are an organism of cells (75 Trillion+) our cell membrane health is of vital importance.

When you eat fat, it is then digested and broken down into fatty acid molecules differing in length, your brain then uses these materials to form special types of fat which it incorporates into its cell membranes.

The specialised brain cells called neurons are contained with a thin double layer of fatty acids.

A protective sheath known as myelin covers the neurons and it is made of of 70% fat.

A big part of myelin comes from one of the most abundant fatty acids found in our body, oleic acid. Great sources of fatty acids include almonds, pecans, avocados and macadamia nuts.

You are also able to get fatty acids from foods such as salmon, sardines, mackerel, walnuts, flax seeds and green leafy vegetables. This is why some people call fish "brain food".

The best source of some fatty acids come from oils, flaxseed and canola oil are good sources.

Another vital source of fatty acids for our bodies and one many people in the UK MISS OUT – is OFFAL.

Yes offal, internal organ meat, it's gone out of fashion in recent years. Offal contains high levels of phospholipids. Phospholipids are fatty acids and are found in every cell throughout the body.

All these foods will allow your brain to absorb and process information more effectively and efficiently and give you better clarity and concentration.

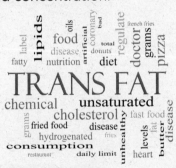

How Trans Fats Effect Our Brain

Trans fats have a very different effect on our brain compared to the other fats I have mentioned – in fact it's a totally opposite effect to the fatty acids.

Trans fats are made in the lab not by nature which means that our body is not used to, doesn't recognise and cannot cope with regular consumption of these fats.

Trans fatty foods such as chips, margarine, biscuits and crisps that contain hydrogenated oils, disrupt communication in your brain.

By constantly eating these types of food we are weakening our own brain, dumbing ourselves down, as well as all of the other negatives associated with eating these types of foods.

The trans fatty acids get into the brain through cell membranes and cause cellular degeneration as well as reduced mental performance.

Our brain cells function by having a certain degree of flexibility, which allows them to maintain a balance alongside different fatty acids in our cell membranes.

Trans fats make the brain cells tight and rigid and reduce its function.

So stock up on good quality fat boosting foods, and you will allow your brain the freedom to function as wonderfully as it is supposed to.

Butter V Margarine

Did you know? If you place a small piece of butter and margarine outside on a plate, the butter will get eaten by ants and the margarine will not get touched. It's classified as a non food, and doesn't really need to be in the fridge in Tesco's!

So it's not good enough for the ants but it's good enough for us, what do they "instinctively know" that we don't?...

Factoid number 2 - Margarine is classified as a non-food!

Historically it was always margarine v butter and the margarine manufacturers would say butter was unhealthy due to the saturated fat. Now butter is having a come back, the margarine manufacturers have actually started to ADD butter to their man made junk. I would always recommend eating real butter.

CHAPTER SIX

What You Need To Know About Protein?

Old Rule: High protein diets are good for fat loss and muscle maintenance.

New Rule: High animal protein diets need to be tailored to make sure they are healthy over the long term.

Over the years my thoughts and choices regarding protein have changed greatly.

I used to follow a high protein diet, religiously eating 30-40g of protein every THREE hours, more than 240g a day, which is the equivalent to 6 large Chicken breasts.

I once drank two tins of tuna blended with a pint of water, just to get my protein fix.

The belief was that the protein maintained the muscle and

encouraged the body to lose fat and not hold water, which it did.

High Animal Protein Diet

High levels of animal protein are bad over long term. Cooked animal proteins are also very hard on the digestive system and take lots of energy to break down.

Processing excess amounts of animal protein can put pressure on the kidneys, with excess animal protein being linked with kidney problems.

One of the benefits of the OLD RULES surrounding protein was that it acted as a diuretic, and kept you from holding water, which made you leaner and drop fat.

The trouble was the diuretic effect was due to the kidneys being forced to flush out excess proteins along with water, which can lead to dehydration, thus making you feel weak and tired (which is what happened to me).

Also another important point, the amount of calcium required by the body increases with the amount of protein consumed, therefore, if your body is unable to get the minimum required calcium, it will start taking out calcium from your bones in order to process the protein.

This can lead to osteoporosis, where the bones tend to become brittle and break easily.

If you eat a high animal protein diet you will see an increase in inflammation, which as you will learn in the following chapters, is a big NEGATIVE.

As we have already discussed inflammation contributes to a number of diseases, such as heart disease, arthritis, diabetes, stroke, and cancer.

While on a high animal protein diet you can become tired and inflamed and it will affect your overall health.

Therefore, it can't be the best long-term approach for fat loss.

I have now learned there are easier ways AND TASTIER ways to achieve the same outcome.

There is only so much cooked meat you can digest and absorb, plus protein can be quite expensive, and it's a shame to WASTE money.

If you have been following a high animal protein diet for more than 9 months you would benefit from a decrease in cooked food intake and an increase in raw food intake.

Even if you continue to eat lots of animal protein, the first thing to do is to increase your raw food intake if you eat more meat, this will help your body digest the meat more easily.

My advice is to have time away from meat, for at least one or two days a week, in fact have some time away from food all together (see chapter Six on fasting), it will do you good.

Try to include more raw food such as salads and steamed vegetables in your weekly food plan.

You can still have a moderate to high protein intake but as well as animals as a source of protein, it should include vegetable proteins as well.

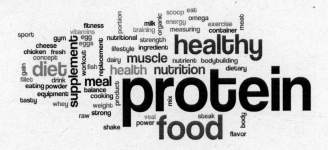

The general guidelines I follow now are to eat protein or a nourishing meal, every 4-6 hours instead of every 3 hours, it's SO much easier than the OLD RULES and improves overall body FAT levels as good if not better than following the OLD RULES.

Trust me when I say your muscles won't decimate and wither away like I used to believe, so long as generally speaking, you have two or three meals that contain protein most days, animal or vegetable.

Vegetable proteins are found surprisingly in vegetables such as beans, legumes and pulses, also there are vegetable proteins in brown rice and peas.

I use a veggie protein powder that contains pea, hemp and rice protein.

- The biggest benefits from a plant-based diet are:

- Raw food is good for you because of the enzymes contained inside them help the body to digest the meal

- Plant based diets are great at reducing inflammation levels in the body.

- When you eat more raw foods, digestive problems can often go away (because of the prebiotics found in vegetables).

Top Tip: Eat beef, cooked as rare as possible, as it is easier to digest the less cooked it is.

CHAPTER SEVEN

Is Salt Bad For You?

**Old Rule: Salt is BAD for you and
increases your blood pressure.**

**New Rule: Salt is OK in the right quantities and
the right type.**

Is salt really bad for you? Just like saturated fat, salt has a very bad reputation.

Just like saturated fat, salt is actually needed in the body for it to work optimally.

Salt is not totally harmless, but it's not the devil in disguise either.

Confused? Most people are.

Basically our body needs salt but at the same time research has proven that too much of it can also be bad for us.

Today I will explain why this confusion has arisen and what you need to know and what you can do about it.

I will provide you with some solutions to help you avoid the negatives and gain all the positives to be had from salt.

Firstly let's have a quick look into the history of salt and find out how it got such a bad name for itself.

How Salt Got its Bad Name

There was one big study carried out in the 1980s called 'Intersalt', this study aimed to find out if there was a relationship between high blood pressure and salt intake.

The study showed a very small link between the two.

It was found that some undeveloped non industrial people who had very low salt intake were found to have low blood pressure.

The leaders of the study were happy with this and used this as proof that if a low salt diet gave low blood pressure then high salt diet must result in high blood pressure.

But then there was another group in the study who mucked up the results and put the first "result" into question.

This was a tribe called the Kuna from Panama.

It was again found that they had low blood pressure and low salt intake.

They decided to test their hypothesis further by increasing the salt intake of the Kuna, sometimes up to 6 teaspoons a day.

The result was there was no change in the hypertensive statuses (blood pressure) of the tribe, no matter what age they were.
(http://www.ncbi.nlm.nih.gov/pmc/articles/PMC1834069/)

However these days it's widely accepted, it's been proven over and over, if you drastically cut your salt intake there probably will be a slight drop in your blood pressure.

This drop is mostly due to the immediate drop in body weight that you get when you cut out salt.

But there is a lot of evidence to suggest that although salt reduction can lead to slightly lower blood pressure all out salt reduction can also lead to health problems.

A study in 2011 showed that after 7 days on a low salt diet in healthy male and female subjects; insulin resistance was increased when compared to a diet high in salt. (Insulin resistance is bad and can lead to hormonal problems and weight gain.)
(http://www.ncbi.nlm.nih.gov/pubmed/21036373)

Another study that was testing the relationship between blood pressure and salt intake found that a reduced salt diet had negative effects on cholesterol levels and stress hormone levels - a sure sign the body is not happy.

This study found that you are more at risk of strokes and heart attacks if you eat under 3 grams of sodium a day than you are when you eat 6-7 grams of sodium a day.
(http://www.sciencedaily.com/releases/2011/11/111123132935.html)

There is a lot of evidence to suggest that salt is OK when eaten in the right form and the right amounts.
Salt has been used as a bit of a scapegoat by health and nutrition experts who suggest that salt causes obesity, high blood pressure and countless other health problems.

Most of the salt in a western type diet (ours) would come from salt "already added" to your foods.

I personally feel that the type of hidden salt in food is worse that the stuff you sprinkle on top of food.

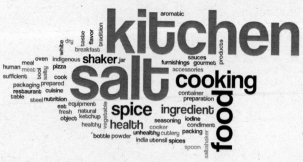

This is where your main focus should be, cutting out these high salt – processed foods.

The best overall indicator of health is ultimately how long you live!

A study found that people with an average salt intake tend to live longer than those who consume too much or too little salt. *(http://eathropology.com/2013/05/21/the-nacl-debacle-part-2-we-dont-need-no-stinkin-science-2/)*

The figure of the average salt intake was just under 2 teaspoons a day.

I personally think salt quality is more important than quantity, and 5-10g of salt per day is OK for the average person.

I also believe salt intake should fluctuate. For example, it should increase if you sweat or exercise lots, and decrease if you are totally inactive (the same as for food in general, if you do more you need more).

If you, like me, are a salt lover, you will be pleased to hear that there are more benefits.

Salt is good for you when you exercise, it helps to keep you hydrated.

Is Salt Bad For You?

You may have heard about electrolytes, and how, when we exercise, we need to replace them, that's what big brands like lucozade and powerade brag about (you don't need these by the way).

This study has found that if you increase your sodium intake before exercise in warm conditions it increases fluid volume (water in the body) and reduces the physiological strain of the exercise.
(http://www.ncbi.nlm.nih.gov/pubmed/17218894)

This doesn't only apply to hot weather conditions - it works for all sports and conditions. Don't just start taking salt before you train or play – buy some salt tablets or rehydrate powder.

If you eat a low salt diet and you exercise regularly, or are an athlete, I could make a good bet you are not going to be performing at your best.

High-flying corporate clients of mine enjoy being compared to athletes. Their performance in their job would also be diminished on a low salt diet.

Being at your best physically and mentally is essential if you want to progress in your job and secure better earnings for the future.

A little story about a good school friend of mine Dean Llewellyn, who is an Ironman competitor.

Dean was competing in his biggest, most difficult and most important race up to that point – Lanzarote Ironman. (Ironman triathlon distance, for those who don't know, you have to complete a 2.4 mile swim, 112 mile bike ride and run a full marathon (26.2 miles) to finish).

Unfortunately, as he was nearing the finish line, literally in the last mile, he collapsed and went into a coma. He told me he remembered thinking he had been run over by a car.

It turned out he had suffered hyponatremia – which is a condition caused when there is not enough sodium (salt) in the body fluids.

Firstly we couldn't figure out how or why it had happened. His race prep had been perfect and then he realised. During the 4 or 5 days of his pre race preparation, he drank loads of water. I mean loads.

The strategy was partially correct as Lanzarote is a hard Ironman because of the hot weather conditions.

The trouble is when you drink loads of water you actually flush the salts out of your body. We now firmly believe that's what Dean had inadvertently done.

Lesson learned. He went back a couple of years later and completed the course successfully. He is a hell of a guy, really tough man and has overcome many challenging injuries since.

Salt Makes Food Tastier

This is one of the big ones for me!

I admit that vegetables and salad can taste boring on their own, but drizzle with some extra virgin olive oil, vinegar, and add some salt and pepper and you have a completely different tasting meal.

Same as kale – delicious with salt and oil – bitter without it.

I believe we should enjoy our food, and not many people will be able to stick to a flavourless diet, I know I can't.

Salt does make a whole world of a difference to food so use it, if adding salt to your veg or salad helps you to avoid unhealthy dressings and sauces then do it, it's a lot better for you.

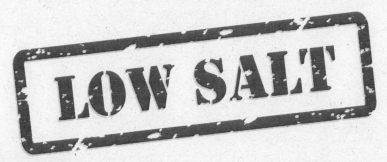

Types Of Salt

After getting the quantity of salt correct, next is the quality of salt.

Often people make no distinction between the different types of salt – BIG mistake.

Some salts are a lot better than others.

There are basically three different types of salt we eat:

1. Sodium Chloride – This is the normal table salt that you get. This is the kind of stuff contained in all of the crap processed foods, it's toxic and it's bad for your health. This is the salt that gave salt as a whole a bad reputation! It's been heated to 400 degrees, bleached, stripped of most of its nutrients during the refining process and has lots of chemicals added to it. It's as far from salt as salt can get.

I personally find table salt and salt from the chippy (yes I eat chips on occasion!) – very strong salty taste (which is lovely and very more-ish) compared with the salt I now use at home which is dead sea salt.

2. So called 'sea salt' – This should be good for you but unfortunately it has been processed and refined so much that it has lost so many valuable minerals that often it isn't much better than the normal table salt mentioned above.

47

Unprocessed salt contains: Calcium, Copper, Iodine, Iron, Manganese, Magnesium and Zinc.

Processed salt does not contain the same nutrients in the same quantities, they are mostly stripped away by the processing.

3. Celtic sea salt – This is the salt that you should be eating. It is sometimes known as 'macrobiotic, hand harvested, sun dried sea salt'. This is real salt and this is what we need, this will help us achieve optimal health. It contains no additives and nothing has been removed which would alter the salt.

You can try to use organic unrefined sea salt or something similar.

Celtic sea salt has been found to help regulate heartbeat and blood pressure, improve brain function, balance blood sugar, alkalise and energise the body and promote sleep. Not bad for something you sprinkle on your food to boost the flavour.

As I have told you in the past, our bodies are made up of a community of cells.

Salt is contained in every single one of these trillions of cells, if it wasn't important I don't think that it would be in every cell.

Every time we sweat, cry or go to the toilet we lose salt, so it is important that these are replaced.

So don't believe everything bad about salt and don't be put off.

It's all about quality and quantity.

As long as you have the right types of salt in the right amounts you can experience many benefits. If you sweat lots because of exercise or in hot weather, remember you need more.

CHAPTER EIGHT

IT'S THE MOST IMPORTANT MEAL OF THE DAY...ISN'T IT?

Old Rule: Skipping meals will slow your metabolism and breakfast is the most important meal of the day

New Rule: Missing meals in the short term actually speeds up your metabolism.

Ok, just like the other rules, this rule was a big part of my approach for many years.

As I told you in the previous chapter, I used to eat every three hours, up to six meals a day and I was in decent shape, but it was HARD WORK and made me ill in the end.

It made me tired and sluggish and nutrient depleted because it was "chicken/steak/eggs, rice and mixed veg" for every meal, every day, for years.

This approach was based on the premise that eating regularly speeded up your metabolism.

Conversely if you skipped a meal your metabolism would slow down.

We thought that if you could boost your metabolism you would in turn lose more fat.

Based on that, breakfast would be the most important meal of the day for weight loss. Again all very logical.

Turns out that it takes a lot more than skipping breakfast or a few meals to slow your metabolism.

In fact research suggests that it can take anywhere from 60-96 hrs of starvation to affect your resting metabolism, and its suggested that even then it would only drop by 8-10%.

Other research has said the opposite is true.

After two and a half or three days (or more) in starvation they saw an INCREASE in metabolism.
*(http://www.ncbi.nlm.nih.gov/pubmed/2405717;
http://www.ncbi.nlm.nih.gov/pubmed/10837292)*

So if fasting actually has some benefits, what are they?

1. A reduction in circulating blood sugars
2. A reduction in insulin levels
3. An increase in growth hormone, which despite its name helps weight loss
4. Improves insulin sensitivity (this also helps weight loss)
5. Increases energy (via catecholamines such as epinephrine and norepinephrine)

Some of those benefits are also gained from just skipping a meal or two.

Fasting Diet Plans

These are diet plans that involve controlled structured fasting, and can really give fat loss a huge boost.

How to do it...

18-24hrs Fast. If you have overeaten, the next day CUT BACK, it's a simple, yet effective strategy.

Try fasting in the morning - drink plenty of water, and dont eating anything until lunchtime or preferably dinner.

I also like to use hot water and lemon as it cleans my gut and restores my body to normal quickly.

You may have heard of the 5:2 diet or variations of it, its what's called intermittent fasting.

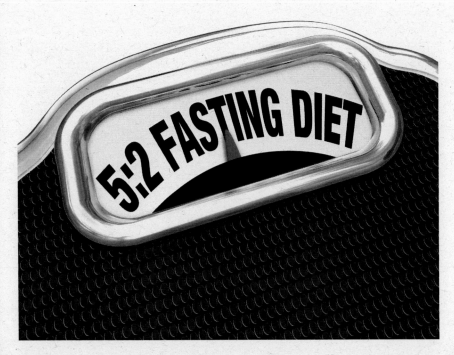

Skip breakfast and eat low calorie or 1-2 light meals a day for 2 non-consecutive days and eat normally for 5 days.

Due to the progressive nature of us as humanoids this has now of course been progressed to 4:3 and even 2:5 or in other words, 2 light meals a day for 5 days and eat normally (whatever that is) for 2 days.

Fasting is a good tool but don't over do it. Listen to your body and be sensible.

Exercise is also an effective tool when used in conjunction with intermittent fasting. I'm not saying to starve yourself and train your ass off, but light exercise with a lean diet will give you good results, but again be sensible.

Just like fasting, exercise increases lots of the good hormones and reduces most of the bad ones.

CHAPTER NINE

Toxins - Why Your Fat Cells May Be Broken

Old Rule: Additives and preservatives are all safe, and in the levels found in food have no ill effects on the human body.

New Rule: Toxins like additives and preservatives are stored in the body, disrupt our hormones and bad for our health.

What we now know is toxins cause havoc in our bodies, clogging up the membranes of our fat cells, disrupting our hormones and causing illness such as allergies and diseases such as cancer.

All these toxins are made from PETROCHEMICALS. These chemicals are originally derived from CRUDE OIL.

The next time you rub that moisturiser on or spray that perfume (gents) remember its crude oil you are rubbing on your body and whatever you put on your skin you absorb.

You end up consuming gallons of these "beauty products" through your skin each year.

Are Your Fat Cells Broken?

There are said to be over 200 non-human chemicals found in the umbilical cord of an unborn baby and hundreds more in our water supply.

Men are now developing breast tissue because of estrogen and women are developing facial hair because of testosterone.

Children as young as 5-6 years old are starting their menstrual cycles and developing breasts.

Toxins are removed from your system by your liver. When toxins are high your liver is overwhelmed, it can't do its job.

Then, toxins in our food and environment are pushed back into the bloodstream and then are absorbed by the fat cells.

Long term, high levels of pesticides and other toxins means the body will have to create additional fat to absorb the toxins – "to mop up the waste".

As the fat cells that are there are already full up.

These toxins can be stored for many years and cause oxidation/Inflammation (free radical damage).
The toxins are stored in the cell membrane and the membrane becomes tough and impermeable causing fat loss to be more difficult.

A growing body of evidence suggests that even when people consume the same amount of calories, a person eating an oganic style diet will lose around 1/3 more weight over 12 weeks than their counterpart who is eating a diet containing pesticides.

Could You Be Weight Loss Resistant?

Other areas of research have compared different groups group of dieters (lean & obese), and tried them on a variety of diets and exercise regimes, to see how they responded.

The major outcomes have been that the people who could not lose weight had the presence of high levels of toxins in their fat cells, (PCBs & pesticides), whether they were lean or obese.

From the many thousands of possible sources of toxins that affect us there are THREE main sources of toxicity that effect us every single day:

1. Food & Drinks that we consume
2. Air & Water
3. Personal Products we put on our bodies

Our supermarkets are filled with food that has a nutritional value of cardboard.

Foods which are packed with chemicals, preservatives, sugars and fats just to make them 'tasty' and more importantly convenient for us to eat in today's busy world.

This is the reason why I am such a big advocate of organic food.

The Need To Detox

So with all of these toxins damaging our health what can we do?

A period of detoxification is the best way to start to rid your body of all of these unwanted substances we have been placing into your body.

The main aim of a detox is to cleanse the blood, liver, gut and entire body from harmful toxins

Another bi-product of a detoxification plan is it reduces inflammation and can take the body from being in ACIDIC state to an ALKALINE state (more on both those subjects in the next chapter).

These stored toxins combined with stress can affect your health in very unpleasant ways:
- Weight gain
- Headaches
- Feelings of fatigue and weakness
- Heartburn
- Sore muscles and skin
- Joint pains

A detox will help you to eliminate these symptoms.

Exercise is made even harder when we are toxin rich we have to work a lot harder because we were all ready exhausted before we began. I found a new lease of life with my exercising, post detox.

By ridding your body of these toxins it can jump start all of your organs and give them the license to work to their full potential, leaving us feeling great!

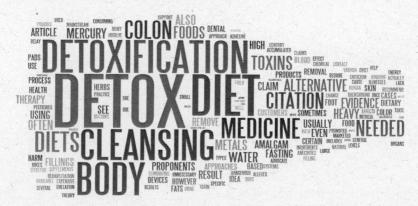

Detoxifications will help rebalance your hormones, reduce your acidity and inflammation levels.

Organic Food

Some of the big benefits of organic eating are:

1. Increased Health – By going organic you don't have to worry about these toxic pesticides harming your health.

2. Nutritionally Stronger Foods – Organic foods are grown differently to non organic foods, it is a more natural process which means that organic fruits and vegetables can contain more than 50% more vitamins, minerals than their non organic rivals.

3. Environmentally and Animal Friendly – Eating this way will also mean that the animals used to produce the food lived a nicer healthier life.

4. Tastier Food – The organic farming methods create healthier animals and plants that gives a much better taste.

The top 18 foods you don't need to eat organic are:

1. Onions
2. Avocado
3. Sweet corn
4. Pineapple
5. Grapefruit
6. Mango
7. Asparagus
8. Peas
9. Kiwis
10. Cabbage
11. Aubergine
12. Papaya
13. Watermelon
14. Cantaloupe
15. Broccoli
16. Tomatoes
17. Sweet potato
18. Mushrooms

(List adapted from the clean 15)

Now I will give you 27 different foods which you should aim to eat organically as these foods are the worst affected by pesticides.

1. Meats (beef, pork, etc.)
2. Fish
3. Milk
4. Butter
5. Eggs
6. Baby Food
7. Peanut Butter
8. Wine
9. Chocolate
10. Apples
11. Coffee
12. Celery
13. Cherry Tomato
14. Cucumbers
15. Grapes
16. Nectarines
17. Peaches
18. Pears
19. Potatoes
20. Hot Peppers
21. Sweet Peppers
22. Strawberries
23. Spinach
24. Kale
25. Courgette
26. Lettuce
27. Blueberries

(Adapted from the Dirty Dozen)

Top Tip: Buy local & seasonal food. If you know that the particular fruit and vegetables are local and are in season then it's a safe bet that the process was a lot more natural. Try going to a local butchers, green grocers or a farmers market for your fresh meat and produce. British standards are still pretty high compared to other countries, but there are constant attempts to dilute these standards.

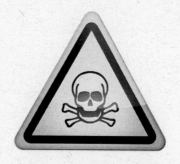

CHAPTER TEN

Inflammation - The Fire Burning Inside You

Old Rule: Saturated fat, smoking and poor lifestyle contribute to and are the main causes of cholesterol and heart disease and related illnesses.

New Rule: Inflammation causes cholesterol to raise and heart disease

Inflammation is very common and reducing it is key to becoming HEALTHY and as I have already taught you, being healthy is the best thing you can do to LOSE FAT.

What is Inflammation?

Inflammation is the body's biological response of attempting to protect itself. It aims to remove harmful stimuli, such as pathogens, damaged cells and irritants; this is the first step of the healing process.

Inflammation triggers a response from the immune system.

Initially inflammation is beneficial for protection, but a lot of the time inflammation can lead to further inflammation that is bad. Most inflammation is acute (short term) and comes from accidents we have when we hurt ourselves, most of the time we recover and heal fully.

Chronic Inflammation

Chronic means long term. Chronic inflammation is when the initial inflammation does not go away and lingers longer than it should. It is no longer an acute healing response but now it's more an indicator that something is wrong.

It is vital to do everything you can to reduce and prevent further inflammation so you don't reach this chronic stage.

Resolution of a chronic inflammatory condition lies at the heart of all attempts to treat and prevent lots of terrible diseases.

One of the biggest causes of chronic disease comes from the presence of 'chronic inflammation'. There are so many diseases and illnesses that are classified as chronic inflammatory conditions:

- Cardiovascular disease
- Diabetes type II
- Metabolic syndrome
- Fibromyalgia
- Chronic fatigue
- Depression
- Alzheimer's disease
- Cancer
- Osteoarthritis
- IBS
- Obesity
- Candida albicans
- Helicobacter
- Atherosclerosis

Inflammatory conditions are often multifaceted and hard to treat.

Cortisol, a stress hormone – is a very powerful anti-inflamatory and is released in response to inflammation and stress. The trouble is, cortisol is similar to insulin in the fact that it is a FAT STORAGE hormone. So, although in the short term it can be useful, in a chronic situation it's not good for weight loss or general health indicators such as sleep.

What causes the inflammation in the first place?

- Chronic infections
- Obesity
- Environmental toxins
- Physiological stress
- Intensive /endurance training
- Physical trauma
- Allergies
- Poor gut health
- Age
- Autoimmune disease
- Lack of sleep

Addressing the above factors will help reduce inflammation greatly.

Inflammation is affecting everything from our livers and bowels to our muscles and joints.

Inflammatory foods, you would be advised to steer clear of include:
1. Processed foods
2. Fast food and Take Aways (especially deep fried foods)
3. Bread (most stuff containing wheat and gluten)
4. All trans-fats/hydrogenated fats
5. Sugar and flour
6. Margarine.

So, what advice can I give you as an alternative diet?

Firstly, eat less junk food and bad fats (like those in fried & processed foods), and take on board more good fats, like extra virgin olive oil, normal butter, coconut oil, avocado, eggs and nuts.

Foods high in Omega-3 fatty acids have been proven to be anti-inflammatory.

Fish is a good source of omega 3s, so stock up on sardines, salmon, herring and anchovies or take a quality fish oil supplement.

Also, use more herbs and spices in your food, such as turmeric, ginger, black pepper, cayenne pepper, basil, chives, cinnamon, parsley and nutmeg as they are all natural anti-inflammatories.

Fruit and vegetables are packed full of antioxidants and vitamins, which are proven to be anti-inflammatory.

Vegetables such as onions, spinach, sweet potato, peppers, garlic, broccoli and other green leafy vegetables are anti-inflammatory as are good fruits such as blueberries, raspberries and strawberries.

Top Tip: Test your level of inflammation. Test it and know your numbers so you can keep an eye on it and try and reduce it. You will need to see your GP for the test or go do it privately (it's called a C reactive protein test or CRP test).

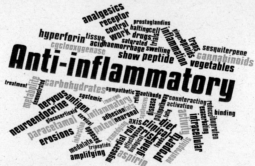

What are the solutions?

Many people who suffer from chronic inflammation do so as a result of their lifestyle, so in order to reduce their symptoms then the lifestyle needs to be changed.

The Fire Burning Inside You Inflammation

Recall the four things that affect our overall health:
1. Acidity
2. Inflammation
3. Deficiency
4. Disease

So if we can: REDUCE acidity levels and FIX any deficiencies.

We will reduce overall INFLAMMATION & hopefully DISEASE.

Let me explain...

If a person was following a poor diet and lifestyle and we firstly fixed that by Cutting Out The Crap (COTC), then that would help reduce acidity and inflammation.

Also, let's say the person was deficient in vitamin D, and you fixed that deficiency with a supplement, the person's inflammation levels would further reduce. In conjunction with general increases in inflammation, the acidity levels inside the body would also increase.

Therefore, if you can reduce the acidity, you can reduce the inflammation and in turn reduce the disease.

Acid & Alkaline

Do you remember back in school, in chemistry lessons, experimenting with those PH strips made of litmus paper?

It used to turn different colours depending on the PH of a solution.

Anyway, you can test your urine or saliva for PH, most people I test are at 5 or 6 and are ACIDIC.

0-6 = Acidic
7-14 = Alkaline

Ideally you would like to be 7.24 ALKALINE.

What is the difference between being acidic and alkaline?

The research suggests that alkaline bodies are able to absorb up to 20 times more oxygen than acidic bodies, also if your body is acidic you are much more susceptible to illness and disease.

Disease thrives in acidity and health thrives in alkalinity.

Dr. Otto Warburg, winner of the 1931 Nobel Prize for his studies in cell respiration, believed that a person's level of health and vitality has a direct correlation to the levels of oxygen in his or her blood stream.

He proved that: diseases can't survive in an oxygenated, alkaline environment.

What determines our acidity or alkalinity?

The main determinant of our body's level of acidity and alkalinity is the foods and drinks we consume.

The more acidic foods and drinks we consume, the higher the levels of acidity. This causes your oxygen levels to drop. This leaves you feeling tired and fatigued.

A western style diet including alcohol, processed foods, caffeine, white carbs and fast foods will make our body more likely to be acidic.

What is the best course of action?

The best course of action to reduce the level of acidity in your body is to remove as many acidic and processed foods as possible and eat a diet high in green vegetables.

By neutralising the acidity your body is much more likely to perform to its full potential.

A detox diet would help, all my diet plans are detoxifying. All detox diets should be alkaline forming.

To speed up the process you can use up to 1tsp of bicarbonate of soda in a glass of water or an easy to get hold of supplement is alkalising salts, and is also a great way of helping you to become more alkaline. Take 1-2 times a day.

As I mentioned the foods we eat have a major effect on whether we are acidic or alkaline so by cutting out these 'bad' foods we will limit the amount of acidity in our bodies.

Some Examples Of Acidic Foods:
- Processed foods, fast food and takeaways
- Omega 6 fats – you can find these in many oils like sunflower oil.
- Bread – most wheat and gluten containing products
- Alcohol
- Coffee
- All trans-fats
- Sugar and flour
- Bacon and sausages
- Margarine

CHAPTER ELEVEN

Cholesterol - Guilty Until Proven Innocent

Old Rule: Cholesterol is essentially undesirable, and is caused by saturated fats, and clogs our arteries.

New Rule: Cholesterol, in the main is important for normal functioning and beneficial, low levels are dangerous.

The Big Cholesterol Con

If the previous chapters have gone against traditional approaches, this one is going totally against what is seen as the norm or the status quo.

So here goes another cracker. Hold on tight, as I don't go gently!

If you have elevated cholesterol and or take statin medication, you need to read this.

It has been drilled into us for the past 50 years that cholesterol is bad for us, so now for someone to say that it is not the case is a bit confusing.

It seems that "guilty until proven innocent" is the case here. Cholesterol has been given a hard time of it, and unfairly so.

Here is the important point and what has changed. So the new school of thought goes like this: cholesterol doesn't cause heart disease, neither do saturated fats – inflammation does.

Let's dig a bit deeper...

Mostly we all think cholesterol is bad for us, this is because it's what we have been told over the last 50 years or more.

Cholesterol is often described as "artery clogging" and is used as an indicator of heart disease, and it is that relationship we will look at today.

Most people believe the less cholesterol they have in their diet the better.

The presumption that cholesterol is bad for you has now been brought into serious question.

Books such as "The Great Cholesterol Myth" explain it in much more detail and I highly recommended if you want the full story.
"Elevated cholesterol is a nonexistent disease" (The Great Cholesterol Myth).

I will explain as simply as possible how and why cholesterol is NOT as bad as you may have been led to believe.

Virtually every cell in the human body can make cholesterol. Most of the cholesterol found in your body is made by the liver and has NOT come from the food you eat.

Important bile acids, vitamin D and steroid hormones (sex

hormones) are all derived from cholesterol.

Cholesterol you would think is therefore essential and reducing it would logically affect other areas, if it were SO important.

However as you probably know, billions of pounds are made selling drugs that will reduce cholesterol, called statins. You may take a statin if your doctor has identified "high cholesterol".

In more recent years, the use of statins has not only being brought into question, but some doctors (especially in the US) will not prescribe them anymore.

About Cholesterol

Cholesterol is a waxy substance that is an important part of our cell membranes (we have around 75 trillion cells in our bodies).

It is also believed that our livers have a natural feedback mechanism that regulates cholesterol production in response to our diet. When we eat more, it makes less, and when we eat less it makes more.

Cholesterol travels around the body as lipoproteins, the most common being high density lipoproteins (HDLs) and low density lipoproteins (LDLs).

Top Tip: If your brain can't handle all the HDL and LDLs letters which appear in the following few paragraphs, just read the last two lines before the subtitle - Arterial Walls. They are the take away points, not all this biochemistry stuff (although I do find it interesting).

The traditional approach to cholesterol and the design of the drugs to treat it, believed that LDLs were the bad guys and HDLs were good and acted as "scavengers", they ate LDLs.

This approach is now thought to be a bit too simplistic and outdated, although not totally off the mark.

The doctors measure a ratio, and the aim was to have more good cholesterol (HDL) than bad cholesterol (LDL). Eating good fats like nuts, seeds, avocado and olive oil are believed to keep HDL levels high. This is still partially true; we now put more importance on the cholesterol profile (we now know there are more types than initially thought).

You can increase HDL by doing some cardiovascular exercise for 30 minutes, such as brisk walking, jogging, cycling or swimming.

More recently the research has suggested that HDL levels are controlled much more by genetic factors than LDL levels. It's also been found that not all HDL is the same. You have HDL-2 and HDL-3, and HDL-2 is more protective and HDL-3 is more inflammatory.

The research still agrees on one thing, having high HDL levels is desirable - although there is now thought to be bad HDL as well as good, just to confuse us ;-).

Initially we thought LDL was bad. Now it's being suggested that it's only bad under certain conditions.

Things are changing fast.

As with HDL, LDL research has moved on. We now have LDL-A and LDL-B.

LDL-B is related to plaque formation and heart disease. High LDL-A is most desirable. Blood tests can now measure ALL these different kinds of cholesterol.

The doctors are able to give you a cholesterol ratio, which indicates the ratio of good to bad cholesterol; research suggests this sort of profile view is still a good indicator of heart disease, much better than total cholesterol alone. Research has suggested that LDL cholesterol is not harmful unless it is damaged.

Arterial Walls

Damaged (oxidised) cholesterol sticks to the lining of the arteries and the process of inflammation begins.
This process is repeated many times and that's the mechanism by which our arteries become clogged and plaques are formed.

The fastest way to damage or oxidise your LDL cholesterol is to SMOKE.

This is why smokers WITH elevated LDL levels are at highest risk of developing heart disease. (It's linked to the production of free radicals by cigarette smoke.)

It should be noted where I live in South Wales, UK, we are a nation of smokers – 23% of Welsh people smoke. The carcinogens in cigarette smoke create lots of free radicals, and that's why smoking is thought to be the biggest causes of oxidised cholesterol, and thus THE greatest risk factor for a coronary event or heart disease.

The latest research by the British Heart Foundation has uncovered yet another type of LDL cholesterol, MGmin-low-Odensity-lipoprotein, which is more common in people with type 2 diabetes and in the elderly, it's "stickier" than normal LDL, which makes it more likely to attach to the artery walls and lead to clogged arteries.

It's been referred to as the "ultra bad boy" and is said to be created by Glycation, a process which happens when there is too much sugar in the blood stream.
The excess sugar is said to "clog up the process" and insert

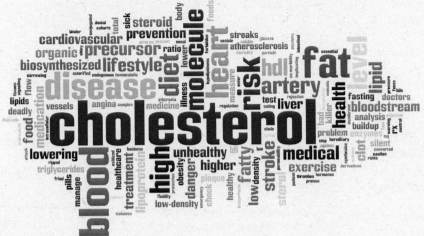

itself where it doesn't belong, in the LDL molecule.

We are continually learning.

First there was just cholesterol, then there were two types, and now there are three or four types. As time goes on our understanding is improving, so we must keep an open mind and a close eye on this topic over the coming years.

One thing that has been proven is that low cholesterol leads to:

• Depression
• Aggression
• Cerebral hemorrhages
• Loss of sex drive.

Now who wants that lot?

History

It all started with the "lipid hypotheses" in the 1950s. A man called Ancel Keys PhD concluded through his studies that excess cholesterol caused heart disease.

Initially he thought that dietary fats drove up cholesterol, but over time, he came to believe that it was saturated fat that drove up cholesterol, and ultimately caused the heart disease.

"The lipid hypothesis has never been proven. Despite 50 years of trying."
(Bowden & Sinatra, The Great Cholesterol Myth, 2012)

BUT, this is exactly what I was taught when I did my degree, and what I believed up until around 2008. This is what many doctors and health practitioners STILL believe today.
The cholesterol research was unable to prove the lipid hypothesis, but what the research did do was hugely improve the knowledge of how cholesterol works.

Thanks to all the research (funded by the drug companies), good and bad cholesterol molecules were identified, and drugs to treat the bad and help the good were developed. People made lots of money.

Anyone who has had high cholesterol (or worked with people who do) for more than 15 years, would have seen various changes (lowering and lowering) in what the "target" figure for someone's cholesterol should be for the best. It is thought that the researchers jumped the gun.

Advisory Group BS - Advisory groups (paid by the drug companies), were set up to encourage the government to keep lowering the safe target for cholesterol levels, so people would have to take more of the statin meds.

Logic

The apparent reason for all the focus on cholesterol is ultimately to make sure we don't get heart disease and die too early.

They even tell people to eat a special diet to keep your cholesterol under control; the diet advised is LOW FAT, HIGH CARBOHYDRATE.

The 5 decades of seeing the results have shown us that the recommended diet does not deliver what it promises, in fact, quite the opposite.

The low fat, high carbohydrate diet, which is also given to diabetics, has failed catastrophically.

Statin Research - Studies that are worth mentioning

The 2008 ENHANCE study, looked at the effectiveness of a combination cholesterol lowering medication called Vytorin. The research project was huge.

The results received lots of negative attention. The new "wonder drug" lowered cholesterol better than a standard statin drug, so you would think they would be happy.

Unfortunately not.

Although people taking the drug saw their cholesterol levels drop like a lead balloon, they still had more plaque growth than the people on the standard version of the drug. The patients on Vytorin also had thicker arterial walls, something which won't help reduce heart disease.

So in a nutshell, their cholesterol went down but their risk for heart disease went up. They still released the drug by the way.
(http://www.nejm.org/doi/full/10.1056/NEJMoa0800742)

Another notable study in the book is Harvard University's "Nurses Health Study", one of the longest running studies of diet and disease ever undertaken. The study followed over

120,000 females since the 1970s to try and determine the risk factors for cancer and heart disease.

In an exhaustive analysis of 84,129 of these women, published in The New England Journal of Medicine, FIVE factors were identified that significantly lowered the risk for heart disease.

The authors wrote "82% of coronary events in the study could be attributed to lack of adherence to these five factors."

1. Don't smoke
2. Drink alcohol in moderation
3. Engage in moderate to vigorous exercise for at least half an hour a day on average.
4. Maintain a healthy weight (BMI under 25)
5. Eat a wholesome low Glycemic (sugar) diet with plenty of omega 3 fats and fibre.

(http://www.channing.harvard.edu/nhs/?page_id=197)

Cholesterol causes heart disease – BULLSHIT!

Dietary cholesterol does not affect cholesterol in the blood, as initially thought.

"When the national cholesterol education programme lowered the optimal cholesterol levels in 2004, eight out of the nine people on the panel had financial ties to the pharmaceutical industry."
(The Great Cholesterol Myth, 2012)

So If Cholesterol Isn't The Cause Of Heart Disease, What Is?

The main cause of heart disease (and many other diseases) is INFLAMMATION. Free radicals production precedes the inflammation.

Raised cholesterol is now thought of as an inflammation problem.

So it is believed that the aim for doctors should be to reduce inflammation rather than reducing cholesterol, and one doctor believes in the future you will have specialist doctors in inflammation.

So in a nut shell...

Free radicals are caused by many things which stress the body, such as food, stress, environmental pollution, smoking, heavy metals (mercury; calcium; aluminium; lead; chlorine; iron; cadmium), too much sunlight, chemicals and pesticides, petroleum based products (women's beauty products), toxins in the home.

Free radicals then wreak havoc in your cells destroying everything they come into contact with.

Long term exposure to free radicals causes oxidation. This oxidation causes the cholesterol in the body to become damaged.

Damaged cholesterol sticks to the lining of the arteries, and the process and cycle of inflammation begins.

Over the long term this can lead to the formation of plaques and atherosclerosis.

Based on this, it has been said, blaming cholesterol for heart disease is like blaming a fire on the firemen who put it out.

Just because the cholesterol is at the site of the problem it does not mean it causes the problem (free radicals and oxidative stress did).

The most important point is that inflammation comes in two types like I have mentioned – acute and chronic.
"Acute inflammation hurts, chronic inflammation kills" (The Cholesterol Con).

Solutions

1. Less sugar and carbs - One important stimulus for the production of cholesterol by the liver is the hormone insulin, which is secreted in response to carbohydrates such as sugars and starch. Dr Briffa says "I have seen many individuals get good control over cholesterol by going easy on their consumption of bread, potatoes, rice and pasta."

2. No Smoking (& moderate alcohol consumption) - The fastest way to damage your cholesterol is to SMOKE. This is why smokers WITH elevated cholesterol levels are at highest risk of developing heart disease.

3. Exercise - has been shown to raise HDL levels, 30 minutes of cardio is fine to get an effect.

4. Good fats - Eating plenty of oily fish such as salmon, mackerel, herring, trout and sardines seems to help raise HDL levels.

5. Nutrition - An anti-inflammatory diet that is high in antioxidants (to blast the free radicals) and high in good sources of fat (to act as an anti-inflammatory).

CHAPTER TWELVE

Hormones

Old Rule: We were not really aware of the role of hormones in fat loss 20 years ago.

New Rule: We now have to be very aware of the role our hormones play and what things can cause them to become out of balance.

I will be trying to keep this stuff as simple as possible as it's a complicated subject, I will share with you how I understand it and apply it to fat loss.

Things That Affect Your Hormones

Foods & Toxins

Junk foods, as mentioned in earlier chapters, have a knock on effect on our hormones, in particular estrogen.

Junk foods contain chemicals which are grouped into a category called Endocrine Disruptors (ED) and they do what they say, disrupt your hormonal balance.

Eating a typical diet high in carbohydrates increases insulin.

Eating FAT actually helps you build new hormones and cholesterol and acts as an anti-inflammatory.

Sleep

If you don't sleep very well it knocks your hormones out of whack, also the opposite is true, if your hormones are out of whack you may not sleep very well.

Either way poor sleep increases: cortisol & leptin, and decreases: testosterone, growth hormone & ghrelin

Stress

Stress, whatever the type (physical, mental or environmental) or cause, in general terms, increases the stress hormone cortisol.

Hormones That Affect Fat Loss

1. Ghrelin
2. Cortisol
3. Insulin (which we have discussed already)

Ghrelin

Ghrelin causes you to feel hungry. Leptin causes you to feel full or satisfied once you have eaten enough. They work opposite from each other in a broad sense.

High levels of Ghrelin hormone can result in uncontrollable food cravings where you will not be satisfied until you have eaten. And higher levels of Leptin hormone will make you stop eating.

High ghrelin levels can lead to fat gain whether you eat or not, so the solution is to reduce your ghrelin levels.

Good news though there are a couple of way to fix your hormones. The first one is easy to do for some... sleep! (And the second one is to eat good high density nutrition foods).

A regular sleeping pattern will dramatically reduce the levels of ghrelin, establish normal levels of Leptin, reduce cortisol and reduce insulin levels.

Aim for 8-10 hours and you'll be fine. Don't try and counter it with 5 cups of coffee in the morning or red bull during the day, just get as much sleep as possible and stick to 1-2 coffees a day max.

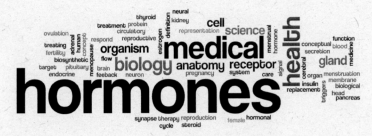

Cortisol

Higher cortisol is directly linked to increased body fat, particularly in the belly area. High cortisol levels increase cravings for carbohydrates and sweet things, which will ultimately lead to gaining body fat.

High cortisol levels can also lead to the body breaking down muscle tissue to use for energy, this will lower what's called your active mass (aka metabolism) and that will ruin your fat loss potential.

The more abdominal fat you have means more cortisol is released, which makes up a very vicious fat gaining circle!

It seems all roads lead to the same destination – weight gain caused by stress messing up our hormones.

So we need to lower our stress levels.

By going to a quiet area, relaxing and trying some deep breathing exercises, which take less than a minute, you can reduce your cortisol levels massively.

Laughing and smiling immediately reduce your cortisol levels.

So the key to success is to attempt to stay as stress free as possible, sleep well and eat well. This will help you beat the cravings and keep your hormones in check.

We all know the great feeling of waking up from a great night's sleep - it gives you the perfect start to the day. We've also all felt sluggish for the whole day after a bad night's sleep, so we need to make sure we are getting enough sleep in our lives.

Getting less than 6 hours a sleep can not only leave us feeling tired and unable to function properly for the day but is bad for your health.

Here are some other benefits of a good night's rest:

- Reduces stress
- Makes you more alert
- Bolsters your memory
- Helps you lose weight
- Reduces depression
- Helps the body repairs

If you want to lose weight it's much easier if you are able to sleep well.

A lack of sleep impacts on the balance of your hormones which then affects your appetite.

A good night's sleep will give you a better balance of all your hormones but specifically your stress and appetite hormones which will help you in your weight loss efforts.

So try and get around 8-10 hours sleep a night, and get your day off to a good start by being full of energy.

Food, Toxins & Hormones

As we discussed in the earlier chapters on food groups (carbohydrates, proteins and fats) and toxins, our food intake and toxic chemicals, can directly affect our hormones.

Exercise & Hormones
Exercise affects our hormones in many ways also, some good and some bad. We will discuss this in the next chapter.

CHAPTER THIRTEEN

The One Treatment That Makes The Biggest Difference To All Health Problems Is Exercise

Old Rule: The more exercise and the harder and more intense that exercise – the better.

New Rule: More exercise and harder is not always healthier – less can be far more beneficial

The old school of thought toward exercise for fat loss was the more the merrier. Exercise as often as possible and as vigorously as possible to burn more calories and lose more fat.

The term in the industry is "a beasting", and I dished them out for years and still do on occasion.

Firstly, the trouble with this approach is that fat loss does not work like that (we alluded to this in the chapter on calories).

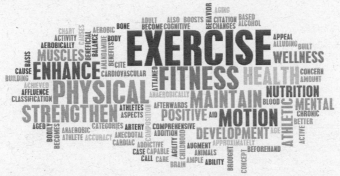

You can't manipulate the calories out (by exercising more) and increase the fat loss exponentially, it only works to a point – "for some of the people for some of the time".

Also the OLD RULE for exercise does not take into account the stress effect that intense exercise has and the long-term effect on joints and inflammation levels in the body.

If intense exercise helped people live longer, then endurance runners and athletes would live the longest, but they don't, they die of heart disease and suffer with joint problems for the last 10 years of their life (generally speaking of course).

People who walk and stay strong by lifting weights (amongst other things) live the longest.

People often don't realize it but intense exercise has a stress effect on the body.

It causes increases in the stress hormone cortisol and it also increases inflammation levels within the body.

So You Should Do less...

One of my clients point blank told me "I hate exercise and everything to do with it".

She had slogged away in the gym for years, and hated every minute of it, and had not seen any real results.

She is not alone. Hating exercise is very common.

The thought of exercise when you are already really tired is very intimidating mentally.

We are in the middle of an energy epidemic, with people drinking more coffee than ever.

The key is the intensity.

Exercising for 20-30 minutes at a higher intensity, two or even three times a week is much better than going twice a week for an hour at a lower intensity.

Although these sessions are "high intensity" they do not have to be high impact or high risk.

My sessions are LOW impact to avoid injury and stress on the joints, as I work mostly with over 40s and 50s.

An interesting 12-week study was carried out in Demark, where moderately overweight males were instructed to expend 300 or 600 calories a day, which is out about 30 or 60 minutes of running.

Both groups were found to lose weight, but interestingly the group which did 60 minutes did not lose any more weight than the 30 minute group (in fact it was slightly less).

Why?

Researchers suggest, firstly, the males who exercised for an hour mentioned they felt tired and said it was very time consuming.

Secondly, the males who exercised for half of the time had a very positive attitude towards exercise and did not find it a burden.

These findings suggest results may be affected by your feelings and perceptions towards the exercise too, so make sure you are enjoying it and are in the right environment and of course getting the right coaching from a good trainer like yours truly.
(http://www.ncbi.nlm.nih.gov/pubmed/22855277)

Do you feel stressed out when you think about exercise?

Feel under pressure to train, but too exhausted to do so?
If you do, it could be affecting your results.

Our body responds to what it needs, not what you think it should have.

Rest is so important, and alongside clean eating, it should form the main part of your journey to reclaim your health, and ultimately get better results for all your efforts.

Three months on and the "I hate exercise" lady has been enjoying two 30-minute sessions per week, and lost over 18lbs.

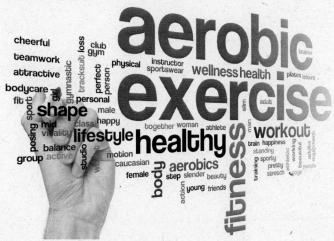

Exercise Enough & You Can Eat What You Want

Some people like to believe this one.

I see so many people 'treating' themselves to rubbish food as a reward for exercising.

Remember you can't out train a poor diet.

Nutrition plays a MAJOR role in shaping your body and exercise plays a MINOR role, I would place about 75% or even 80% of the time working on NUTRITION and only 25% of your time on exercise strategies.

It can be argued that when you exercise regularly you are more focused with your nutrition, if that's the case for you, exercise more often but still 3-4 lots of 30 minutes is enough and mix it between two moderately intense, low impact circuits (remember intensity is relative, its your perception and its relative to your fitness level and experience).

....

Bonus - old exercise related rules, that don't need an entire chapter...

Bonus Old Rule: The fat burning zone is best for fat loss.

Bonus New Rule: It isn't

The fat burning zone strategy is very ineffective. For best fat loss EAT WELL and vary your training stimulus. Mix the speed and intensity and type of exercise to improve results.

Bonus Old Rule: Spot reduction is possible.

Bonus New Rule: It's NOT

Many people still believe the best way to get a flatter tummy would be to do sit ups and to get less fat on your bum do more squats. This is called spot reduction and has been proved to be impossible.

I always use this example – research has shown that a professional, right-handed tennis player does not have any less fat on their right arm than their left, even though they work it a lot more than the left. (They just have stronger muscles). In order to reduce abdominal fat or any other troublesome area you should aim to do whole body exercises not small specific ones.

CHAPTER FOURTEEN

Supplements - Plugging The Hole

Old Rule: You don't need them as you get everything from your food
New Rule: Definitely need them, as we do not get everything from our food

Just to recap quickly from chapter one.

The FOUR reasons the body gets sick:

Acidity
Inflammation
Deficiency
Disease

This chapter will look at why supplements are needed to fill the hole left by malnutrition and deficiencies.

The whole purpose of any supplementation programme is to balance out any deficiencies, and not to take them just for the sake of being "healthier".

As the old and new rules suggest, supplements have become more and more important over the last 60 years.

Supplements

Since the introduction of processed "fake" foods, additives, preservatives and petrochemicals and intensive farming, the food chain has been compromised.

Common Deficiencies/Problem Areas
1. Vitamin D
2. Vitamin C
3. Fish Oils
4. Magnesium
5. Gut Bacteria - Probiotics (acidophilus is recommended)

Supplements can be fantastic for fixing your health if you are lacking in one area. Personally I'm not a lover of oily fish, so I supplement with a quality fish oil.

Supplements are an easy way to make sure you get all of the nutrients you need to stay healthy.

Reasons You Should Take Supplements

Many people's diets leave them deficient. The way some people eat lends itself to deficiency because it's simply not balanced.

They miss out entire food groups such as:
Fish
Vegetables
Meat or Red Meat
Organ Meats
Salt, Herbs & Spices

When you miss out entire food groups it's not gonna help you with your HEALTH and ultimately your FAT LOSS.

Inside your body, generally speaking you have "stores" or "reserves" of nutrients and building materials. They are stored throughout your body, and we can use these stores at any time and take materials we need from places like your blood, bones, muscles and fat.

The reason we need to eat food is to nourish the body and provide it with ALL the BUILDING materials it needs to replenish the stores and work normally.

Many modern foods do the exact opposite. They strip nutrients from your body, making them what's known as ANTI-NUTRIENT foods.

If, like a typical westerner, every meal you eat is TAKING away nutrients from your stores rather than ADDING to them, you will be deficient in some way for sure.

Environment

Modern techniques mean we get fruit that looks great but doesn't always taste great.

Lots of the chemicals and techniques used in intensive farming have taken all the goodness out of the soil.

This also affects the water, we have long known about the effects of acid rain and chemicals from farming and industry getting into our water system.

When plants are repeatedly grown on the same land, the soil loses nutrients faster than they can be replaced.

Farming techniques such as leaving land to fallow have been passed over for modern techniques of spraying the nutrients on top rather than the plant getting them from the soil.

Fertilisers contain just enough nutritents for the plant to survive until harvesting, but not enough to support human health. (Food science makes sure the product looks good).

This result is plants that have up to 75% fewer nutrients.

Supplements

Comparisons of an orange and an asparagus show how things have changed: In the 1940s, one orange provided the same amount of vitamin C as 6 oranges in 2010, and similarly its reported that to get the nourishment of one stick of 1940s asparagus you would now need to eat a whole bunch (6-8 sticks).

In addition to this, most plants sit in stores, on trucks, shelves, and counters for weeks before being eaten.

During that time the nutrient content of these plants FURTHER decreases.

As people age, they often begin taking medications which can also interfere with nutrient absorption.

Exercise also increases your nutrient needs. If you exercise you are using more nutrients for producing energy and to help your body to repair and recover.

Remember you should only supplement if you CAN'T or WON'T eat something.

High nutrient dense foods are always the first choice and supplements would be the last.

However the idea that you can get all your nutrients from food is fine in theory, but virtually impossible in practice.

Soil nutrient depletion, poor unbalanced nutrition and lifestyle, toxins and pesticides, and exercise can all cause nutrient deficiencies.

As a result of all this I believe supplementation, in the right areas, can help you live longer.

SO WHAT ARE THE NEW RULES OF WEIGHT LOSS?

1. Goal: The main goal of your diet and exercise plan should be HEALTH and not fat loss

2. Calorie Intake: All calories are not created equal. The makeup of each calorie is more important than the calorific value itself. We should eat foods with a high density of nutrients inside.

3. Carbs: Carbohydrates need to be closely monitored for fat loss. The higher your body fat generally the less carbohydrates you need. Carbohydrates are activity dependent and your intake should reflect this.

4. Diabetics: It seems that all the anecdotal evidence suggests tht type II diabetics would benefit from following a LOWER carbohydrate diet with a moderate fat intake

5. Fat: Low fat is BAD. Fat, especially saturated fats, are essential for the body, are good for your heart and do not directly affect cholesterol. (see cholesterol chapter)

6. Protein: High animal protein diets need to be tailored to make sure they are healthy over the long term.

7. Salt: Salt is OK in the right quantities and the right type.

8. Metabolism: Missing meals in the short term actually speeds up your metabolism.

9. Chemicals & Toxins: Toxins like additives and preservatives are stored in the body, disrupt our hormones and bad for our health

10. Inflammation: Chronic inflammation and damage from free radicals causes cholesterol to raise and people to develop illnesses such as heart disease, arthritis, diabetes, asthma and cancer, to name but a few.

11. Cholesterol: Cholesterol, in the main is important for normal functioning and beneficial, low levels are dangerous.

12. Hormones: We now have to be very aware of the role our hormones play and what things can cause them to become out of balance.

13. Exercise: More exercise and harder is not always healthier – less can be far more beneficial

14. Supplements: We definitely need to supplement our diet with vitamins and minerals, as we do not get everything we need from our food anymore.

Final Thoughts...

Looking back at the old rules compared to the new I can see such a huge improvement. The new rules consider the wider picture and we have learnt so much over the last 20 years.

That's not to say people didn't have, and still won't have results from the old rules.

However the new rules of weight loss will keep you healthier throughout the journey and allow you to achieve higher levels of weight loss, and it is easier than following the old rules of weight loss.

For many people life seems extraordinarily busy, time is so valuable. Based on that premise, we don't have time to waste.

Life is short and it is wise to invest our time, money and effort in the right areas. Some people have unfortunately already "wasted" lots of their time, money and efforts following the wrong advice.

If through this book I can save you time, and help you get a better return from effort and money you invest, I would have done my job.

I have thoroughly enjoyed researching and presenting these new rules to you. Share this book with your friends and families and help them improve their health.

I hope you have enjoyed the book and have learnt the New Rules Of Weight Loss. If you apply half of what you have learnt you will be well on your way to a healthier and brighter future, whatever life may bring.

If you would like to further progress your weight loss and fitness journey you may want to consider doing my online, 90 day exercise and nutrition programme. The programme is for over 40s and will help you lose weight and get fitter fast. The programme will take you from being totally unfit and hold your hand until you are at a good level of fitness.

Head over to

www.richard-clarke.co.uk

Appendices

Sample Recipes

For a full detailed 14 day plan go here for your free 14 day pass:

http://www.richard-clarke.co.uk/academy/

Breakfasts
Berry & Spinach smoothie (Serves 1)

Ingredients
- 1 handful of strawberries
- 1 handful of blackberries
- 200ml coconut milk or water
- 2 large handfuls of fresh spinach
- Handful of ice cubes

Method
1. Blitz all ingredients in a blender and serve!
2. This is a brilliant way to get more green nutrients!!

Breakfast Courgette Pancakes (Serves 1)

Ingredients
- 1 medium size courgette
- 1 medium size spring onion
- 1 large egg
- Salt to taste
- Pepper to taste
- 2 tbsp coconut oil for frying

Method
1. Grate courgette into a small bowl.
2. Finely chop 1 spring onion and mix with the courgette.
3. Combine 1 large egg into the bowl and mix thoroughly adding salt and pepper to taste.
4. Heat oil in frying pan and spoon 3 mounds of the courgette mixture into the pan and fry until lightly browned, pressing down to flatten. Flip pancake till browned on both sides.

Berries, nuts & full fat Greek yoghurt

Serves 1
Ingredients:
• 2 tablespoon Greek Yogurt or Bio Live yogurt
• Handful of berries
• Small handful of cashew/almond/brazil nuts

Method:
1. Spoon out the yogurt into a bowl
2. Add berries & nuts and mix together
3. Eat immediately

Almond Pancakes (Serves 1-2)

Ingredients
• 1 cup almond flour
• 2 eggs
• 3-4 tbsp of coconut milk
• 1 vanilla pod, split and scraped seeds out
• 1 tbsp of ground cinnamon
• Coconut oil

Method
1. Mix eggs, coconut milk and vanilla in a bowl and whisk together.
2. Sift in almond flour and cinnamon.
3. Heat a large pan over a medium heat; add a tsp of coconut

oil to the pan and add pancake batter in small rounds, quickly turning the pan around to spread the pancake.

4. Cook until brown on the underside, about 45 seconds and then flip to brown other side.

Lunches
Broccoli & Mint Soup (Serves 2)

Ingredients
- 1 large onion, diced
- 1 tbsp coconut oil
- 1 head of broccoli
- 3 cups chicken or vegetable stock
- Small bunch of mint leaves, shredded

Method
1. Fry onion in a large pan with oil on medium heat until softened.
2. Add broccoli and stock and simmer for 10 - 15 minutes or until broccoli has softened. Cool slightly.
3. Place in a food processor with mint leaves or use an electric blender to form a smooth texture.
4. Heat to serve.

Beef Stir Fry (Serves 1)

Ingredients
- 1 organic rib eye steak, cut into strips
- 2 shallots, peeled and chopped lengthwise
- 1 red pepper, chopped into long strips
- 2 garlic cloves, peeled and cut lengthwise
- 4-5 fresh curry leaves
- 1 green chilli, finely chopped
- coconut oil, himalayan rock salt, ground black pepper, ground cinnamon, ground turmeric

Method
1. Mix salt, pepper and turmeric on a plate and cover the beef

strips well with the mix until yellow.

2. Add the shallots, red pepper, garlic, curry leaves, green chilli and a heaped tbsp of cinnamon to a wok or pan with hot coconut oil.

3. Add a little salt and pepper.

4. Cook for about 2 minutes max at high heat and add the beef.

5. Mix it all well and cook beef to taste.

6. Sprinkle a few roughly chopped fresh coriander leaves on top.

7. Serve in a bowl piping hot.

Monkfish & Lemon Skewers (Serves 4)

Ingredients
• 800g monkfish tail fillets, cut into 4cm pieces
• 4 unwaxed lemons
• 2 tsp sumac (see below)
• 1-2 tsp dried red chilli flakes
• Sea salt
• 4 garlic cloves
• A handful of fresh flat leaf parsley, finely chopped
• Salt and freshly ground black pepper
• Wild rocket leaves

Method

1. (Sumac is a blend of spices and is widely used in Turkish cooking. If you can't find it, mix 1 tsp each of lemon zest, toasted crushed cumin seeds and sweet smoked paprika and use this instead)

2. Put the monkfish into a glass bowl. Finely grate the zest of 2 lemons in a separate bowl and set aside. Halve these lemons and squeeze the juice over the fish. Add the sumac and chilli, season well with sea salt and stir. Cover and chill in the fridge for 15-30 minutes.

3. Meanwhile, preheat your grill to high. Add the garlic and parsley to the lemon zest. Season, mix well, and then set aside.

4. Thinly slice the remaining lemons. Thread the monkfish and lemon slices alternatively onto 8 metal skewers (or wooden skewers soaked in water for 30 minutes). Grill for 8-10 min,

turning halfway through, or until the fish is cooked through.
5. Garnish with the zest mixture and serve with rocket salad.

Watercress & Asparagus Soup (Serves 4)

Ingredients
- 900ml of vegetable stock
- 1 small cauliflower – trimmed & roughly chopped
- 350g asparagus spears – trimmed and chopped
- 4 spring onions
- 50g watercress
- 25g fresh mint
- Sea salt & freshly ground black pepper

Method
1. Put the cauliflower in a large pan & bring to the boil. Add the asparagus & spring onions, bringing back to the boil and simmer for 3 minutes.
2. Now take off the boil and stir in the watercress and mint until wilted. Blend the soup in blender or use hand blender and then re-heat and season.

Cauliflower & Coriander Soup (Serves 4)

Ingredients
- 3 tbsp coconut oil
- 1 large onion, finely chopped
- 4 garlic cloves, finely sliced
- 1 1/2 tbsp coriander seeds, roughly ground
- 2 sweet potato, peeled and chopped 1cm cubes
- 1kg cauliflower, leaves discarded washed and sliced approx 1cm thick
- 750ml vegetable stock
- 1 handful fresh coriander, chopped
- 1 tsp chilli flakes

Method
1. Heat a large saucepan over a moderate heat, add the oil, onions garlic, coriander seeds and fry for 10-15 minutes stirring occasionally until golden brown.
2. Add the cauliflower and half the stock then cover and simmer for 20-30 minutes. When the cauliflower and sweet potato are soft add the rest of the stock and continue to simmer for 10 minutes.
3. Using a stick blender or food processor blend the soup to your desired consistency, season and serve or chill and store.

Roasted Tomato Soup

Ingredients
• 2.5kg plum tomatoes (or vine ripe tomatoes)
• 2 tbsp coconut oil
• 1 red onion, peeled and diced
• 1 tsp dried basil
• 1/2 tsp red chilli flakes- if you like heat- or omit
• 1 tin of chopped tomatoes
• 4 yeast free stock cubes, made up
• 1 bay leaf
• Sea salt and freshly ground pepper, to taste

Method
1. What you'll need to do first: Roast the tomatoes.
2. Preheat the oven to 400oF.
3. Cut the plum tomatoes in half and toss them into a roasting pan with the coconut oil, some dried Italian herbs and several peeled cloves of garlic. Add a generous drizzle of lemon juice.
4. Put into the oven and gather the next ingredients. The tomatoes should be ready in roughly 45 minutes.
5. Heat the coconut oil over medium heat. Add the onion and garlic and stir for five minutes. Add the herbs and chilli flakes, and stir for another minute or two, until the onion is softened. Add the canned tomatoes and stock. Toss in the bay leaf and season with sea salt and fresh ground pepper, to taste.
6. Add the oven-roasted tomatoes and garlic, breaking the

pieces apart with a wooden spoon.

7. Cover and bring to a simmer; lower the heat and continue to simmer for about 30 to 40 minutes.

8. Discard the bay leaf.

9. Puree the soup in a blender then return to the pot. Taste for seasoning adjustments. Heat through.

10. If the soup is too thick, add enough hot broth to thin it to the consistency you prefer.

Dinners
Coconut Chicken & Cauliflower Rice (Serves 4)

Coconut Chicken
Ingredients
- 300ml coconut milk
- 2 tbsp tomato puree
- 1 tbsp (or to taste) dried crushed chilli
- 2 tbsp ground almonds
- 2 tsp turmeric
- 2 tsp garam masala
- 2 tsp cumin
- 4 chicken breast fillets, cut into bite size pieces
- 2 onions, chopped
- 2 cloves garlic, crushed or finely chopped
- 2 tbsp Coconut oil
- 4 tbsp fresh coriander

Method
1. Mix the coconut milk with the tomato puree, chilli, almonds, turmeric, garam masala,cumin and 1tbsp water. Add the chicken and coat all of the pieces. Cover with cling film and refrigerate for at least 1 hour
2. Cook the onions and garlic in 1 tsp of coconut oil until soft.
3. Remove the chicken from the marinade, add to the pan with the onion and cook for 2 mins, covered over a low heat. Add the marinade and the remaining oil and cook for 15 - 20 minutes.
4. Stir in the fresh coriander and serve.
Cauliflower rice (serves 4)

Ingredients:
· Head Large Cauliflower (about 250g)

Optional:
· 2 Small Onion
· 2 tbsp Coconut Oil
· 2 tbsp Butter
· 2 Cloves Fresh Garlic
· Freshly Ground Black Pepper

Method (Microwave Recipe)
1. Grate or chop the cauliflower florets to resemble grains of rice.
2. Cook on full power in the microwave for 2 minutes in a lightly covered microwaveable dish (60s if you're just having once portion). No need to add water.

On the Hob Recipe
1. Follow Step One (above)
2. Finely chop the onion and cook in a pan with coconut oil until softened
3. Add the cauliflower and garlic (finely chopped) to the pan and stir well
4. Cover the pan and cook for 5-10 minute or until softened
5. Add pepper and stir in butter if needed.

Chicken In Walnut & Garlic Sauce (Serves 4)

Ingredients
• 4 large chicken breasts, skin removed
• 4 tbsp of coconut oil, melted down
• 3 heaped tbsp of roughly chopped walnuts
• 3 heaped tbsp of chopped parsley
• 3 plump cloves of garlic, peeled and crushed
• Himalayan Sea salt and freshly ground black pepper

Method

1. Preheat the oven to 200°C (400°F) Gas mark 6
2. Place the chicken breasts in an ovenproof serving dish.
3. Put all the remaining ingredients into a food processor and whiz briefly into a sauce.
4. Spread the mixture over the chicken and bake in the oven for 40 minutes until golden and cooked through. Serve with a huge avocado salad.

Sticky Chicken Surf & Turf (Serves 4)

Ingredients
• 2 lemons, quartered
• 12 chicken wings
• 12 uncooked prawns, shell on
• 1tsp oregano
• salt and freshly ground black pepper

For the marinade
• zest and juice of 1 lemon
• 2 tomatoes
• 1 onion
• 4tbsp olive oil
• 1 red chilli
• 6 garlic cloves

Method
1. Preheat oven to 180°C.
2. Put all the marinade ingredients in a blender and whizz till smooth. Throw the chicken into a roasting tin with the marinade and mix to coat. Add the lemon quarters.
3. Roast for 30 minutes, occasionally giving the tray a shake to mix it up.
4. Add the prawns and squeeze the roasted lemons over the ingredients.
5. Cook for a further 10 minutes, or until the prawns are cooked.
6. Serve with a green salad.

Fat loss Fishcake's (Serves 4)

Ingredients
• 1 Rainbow trout
• 100g smoked salmon
• 2 large sweet potatoes
• 1 portion of Soft goats' cheese
• 2 cloves garlic, crushed
• 1 red chilli , diced
• 1 beaten egg
• 6 Chives, chopped finely
• 50g Gluten Free bread crumbs

Method
1. Wrap rainbow trout in foil and place in oven for 25 minutes at 200oc.
2. Once the rainbow trout is cooked, leave out to cool.
3 Peel and boil sweet potatoes, once soft mash and place in a bowl to cool. Flake rainbow trout into the mash, watching out for bones. Cut the smoked salmon into small pieces and add to mash. Then add garlic, chilli and chives.
4. Mix all ingredients together. Place in fridge for 1-2 hours.
5. Now beat an egg in one bowl, Breadcrumbs in another. Remove bowl from fridge. Using your hands take handfuls of mixture and shape into fishcakes. Place the fishcake into the bowl of beaten egg until covered, then into bowl of breadcrumbs until completely covered. Repeat this until you have used all of your mixture (4 fishcakes).
6. Place fishcakes in oven for 30-45 minutes until golden brown. Serve with baby spinach, rocket and cherry tomato salad then drizzle balsamic vinegar and olive oil

Chicken Kebabs (Serves 2)

Ingredients
• 2 Chicken Breast, cubed into 1" pieces
• 1 Yellow Pepper, cut into 1" pieces
• 1 Red Pepper, cut into 1" pieces
• 1 Red Onion, cut into 1" pieces
• 1 Mango, cut into 1" pieces

- 4 Cherry Tomatoes
- Wooden Skewers
- Coconut Oil
- Chilli Flakes

Method
1. Skewer the chicken, onion, pepper, mango and tomatoes onto sticks.
2. Melt coconut oil and brush all over, sprinkle with chilli flakes then grill until the chicken is cooked through.
3. Serve with an avocado salad

Zingy Tuna Steaks (Serves 2)

Ingredients
- 2 x 150g/5oz tuna steaks
- Pinch sea salt
- drizzle extra virgin olive oil
- For the salsa verde
- 1 heaped tsp Dijon mustard
- 150-250ml/5-9fl oz fruity, extra virgin olive oil
- 4 anchovy fillets
- Handful fresh flat leaf parsley
- Handful fresh basil
- Handful fresh tarragon
- 1-2 tbsp capers
- 1 garlic clove
- Pinch sea salt
- 1 lemon, juice only

To serve
- lemon wedges
- 2 sprigs fresh flat leaf parsley and fresh mint

Method
1. Preheat the oven to 200o C/400o F/Gas 6.
2. For the tuna, season the tuna steaks with the sea salt and

drizzle with the olive oil. Rub the salt and oil into the steaks.

3. Heat a heavy-based frying pan until hot. Add a tuna steak to the hot pan and sear until lightly browned. Carefully turn over and sear the other side (this will take about 30 seconds on each side, longer if the tuna is thickly cut). Remove and keep to one side. Repeat with the other tuna steak.

4. Place the tuna steaks in a roasting tray and place in the hot oven for another minute or two (they should still be slightly pink on the inside). Remove and keep warm.

5. For the salsa verde, place the mustard and a few tablespoons of the olive oil in a bowl and whisk to emulsify. Chop the anchovies finely and add to the bowl.

6. Pick the leaves from the herbs (except the basil - you can include the stems in the sauce). Pile the picked herbs onto a chopping board. Sprinkle the capers over the top. Chop the herbs and capers finely with a sharp knife. When finely chopped, add to the bowl with the mustard and oil mixture.

7. Peel the garlic clove. Place it on the chopping board and sprinkle over the sea salt. Crush to a fine paste with a knife blade and add the paste to the bowl and mix. Add some of the remaining olive oil to the bowl. The sauce should have a spooning consistency, so add just enough oil - you may have some left over. Mix thoroughly.

8. Just before serving, add the lemon juice to the sauce (the lemon will cause the herbs to go brown if you add it too early).

9. To serve, place the tuna steaks onto plates. Squeeze over some lemon juice and serve with a wedge of lemon, a dollop of salsa verde and a sprig of parsley each

Big Bad Burger and Chips

Ingredients for Burgers
- 500g extra lean beef mince (or turkey will work fine too)
- 1 onion, chopped finely
- 1 chilli - finely chopped
- 1 x egg

Method

1. Mix all ingredients together in a bowl, divide it into 4 portions. Knead each portion so it all sticks together nicely, then flatten into a burger shape.
2. Heat some coconut oil in a frying pan and shallow fry for around 4 minutes each side.

Ingredients for Wedges

- 2 large sweet potatoes
- 1/2 tsp chilli powder
- 1 tsp paprika
- 1 tbsp coconut oil, melted

Method

1. Slice up the sweet potatoes so they look like wedges.
2. Toss all ingredients into large bowl then place in a large baking tray in oven at around 200-220o C for 30-40 minutes.
3. Serve alongside a bed of steamed greens..

7 Day Diet Plan

	Monday	Tuesday	Wednesday	Thursday	Friday	Saturday	Sunday
Breakfast	Berries, Nuts & Full Fat Greek Yoghurt	Berry & Spinach Smoothie	Berries, Nuts & Full Fat Greek Yoghurt	Berry & Spinach Smoothie	Berries, Nuts & Full Fat Greek Yoghurt	Almond Pancak	Bacon, Eggs, Mushrooms & Tomatoes
Lunch	Choice of Vegetable Soup Watercress & Asparagus Soup	Large Green Salad with Choice of Protein (egg, poultry, fish)	Choice of Vegetable Soup Sweet Potato & Lentil Soup	Large Green Salad with Choice of Protein (egg, poultry, fish)	Choice of Vegetable Soup Roasted Tomato Soup	Large Green Salad with Choice of Protein (egg, poultry, fish)	Choice of Vegetable Soup Broccoli & Mint Soup
Dinner	Sticky Chicken Surf & Turf	Fat Loss Fish Cakes	Chicken Kebabs	Zingy Tuna Steaks	Coconut Chicken Curry	Big Bad Burger & Chips	Any Omelette. Small amount of hard cheese is ok
Snacks	2 Large Celery Sticks	Handful of Berries or and apple	Boiled Egg Salad (1-2 eggs)	30-40g Nuts (almonds, walnuts, brazil)	(have with curry) Cauliflower Rice	Steak & Green Salad	Chicken Drumsticks
Fluids	Water 2-3 litres Coffee x 1 Hot water & lemon	Water 2-3 litres Coffee x 1 Hot water & lemon	Water 2-3 litres Coffee x 1 Hot water & lemon	Water 2-3 litres Coffee x 1 Hot water & lemon	Water 2-3 litres Coffee x 1 Hot water & lemon	Water 2-3 litres Coffee x 1 Hot water & lemon	Water 2-3 litres Coffee x 1 Hot water & lemon

3 Day Exercise Plan

For a full 14 day plan & VIDEOS OF THESE WORKOUTS go here:

http://www.richard-clarke.co.uk/academy/

Day 1

Perform each exercise for either 30, 45 or 60 seconds. Rest between each exercise if needed, and rest after each set of the 4 exercises below are complete.

Squats
Shoulder Press
Sumo Lift
Upright Row
REST

Repeat x 3-5 times

Day 2 - REST

Day 3

Perform each exercise for either 30, 45 or 60 seconds. Rest between each exercise if needed, and rest after each set of the 4 exercises below are complete.

Squats
Shoulder Press
Sumo Lift
Upright Row
Glute Bridges
Crunches

Dorsal raise
REST

Repeat x 2-3 rounds

For a full 14 day plan & VIDEOS OF THESE WORKOUTS go here:

http://www.richard-clarke.co.uk/academy

About

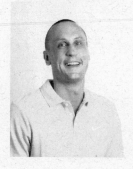

Richard Clarke is an exercise scientist and fat loss specialist from Swansea in South Wales, UK. He helps over 40s and 50s look and feel their best, using his unique, no nonsense approach to exercise and dieting. He provides his health, nutrition & fitness solutions both online at www.richard-clarke.co.uk and at his private gym.

You can find out more about Richard and join his specialist 90-day exercise and WEIGHT LOSS programme online at www.richard-clarke.co.uk

Feel Like You've Been Struggling to Lose Weight Forever?

You've probably been dieting for longer than you can remember.

Your probably just like my clients, and fall off the wagon every weekend.

You're tired and fed up of losing weight and then gaining it all back (and more).

You feel awful and know this cycle just can't go on.

You feel something has to change because this approach is obviously not working.

You're confused and unsure where to turn or what to try next?

It's Not Your Fault...But Does Any Of This Sound familiar?

For many women over 40 losing weight can become a nightmare.

That's why I have transferred my highly successful program ONLINE.

The brand new program allows you to lose weight and get fit in the privacy of your own home.

It's called Weight Loss Forever and closely follows The New Rules Of Weight Loss. It's the perfect solution for anyone who wants to delve deeper and further their learning from what the book has taught.

NOTE: I will personally hold your hand and guide you step by step through 90 days of losing weight and getting fit.

Go here for your FREE 14-DAY PASS:

http://www.richard-clarke.co.uk/academy/

Finally there's:
X No more jumping from diet to diet
X No more short-term fads
X No more desperate strategies like shakes and bars
X No more killing yourself with hours of exercise
X No more stress
X No more confusion
X No more wasting your time

In fact:
✓ Yes you will have fast weight loss
✓ Yes it's a simple system anyone can follow
✓ Yes 1000's of women have already seen results doing it
✓ Yes you will have a long-term, proven strategy
✓ Yes you will be kept motivated so you can keep it off forever
✓ Yes you will have support along the way to keep you on track
✓ Yes I will answer any burning questions you may have
✓ Yes you will get my best-kept weight loss strategies

So here's what you get when you join my 90-Day weight loss and exercise program:

Get my nutrition blueprint for easily losing weight while eating tasty meals and never counting calories. The tasty nutrition plan will help reduce your cravings and sugar intake and leave you feeling full of energy.

I will personally review your food diary and advise you on what THE most important things to change first are, and then help you to change them.

You will have THREE training sessions per week where I will hold your hand and guide you step-by step through your exercises and technique.

Forget dieting and let me show you how to focus on what's really important.

Let me show you how to get over your need for coffee and energy drinks just to get you through the day, and how to boost up your natural energy.

The fitness plan will build you up gradually over the 90 days, introducing you to new exercises each week.

Me teaching you how to do exercises that fix any imbalances and make your body as injury proof as humanly possible.

Ask me questions via live online seminars, called webinars

Watch video tutorials where I will show you exactly how to do everything, and take you through The New Rules Of Weight Loss step by step.

Learn the closely kept secrets that have helped my clients fix their hormones and feel young again.

What you get with the Weight Loss Forever Program again...

1. Workouts. 36 workouts that build you up gradually from a beginner level to above average fitness

2. Nutrition. Meal plans & recipes to help make losing weight easier and more enjoyable.

3. Guidance. Daily prompts to remind you what to do and how to do it

4. Questions Answered. Submit your own questions - ask me anything you want

5. Feedback. Get feedback on your food diaries, plus access to a community of other peoples food diaries and the feedback they have had

6. Tutorials. Watch my weekly educational tutorials where I will teach topics such as carbohydrates and weight loss as simply as possible in 3-5 minutes.

7. Cookbooks. Get four fantastic cookbooks (worth over £50). You cannot even buy THREE of these cookbooks directly as they are exclusively for the weight loss forever clients.

-The first one contains 30 breakfasts, 30 lunches and 30 dinners which all help you lose weight.

-The second one is a SNACKS and TREATS for weight loss cookbook

-The third one is a clean CURRY cookbook.

-The fourth one is a MEAT FREE cookbook for all the vegetarians and people out there who don't want to eat meat all the time.

8. Community. You will get access to a community of like-minded people who are all following the program and losing weight.

9. Lifetime access. You will have lifetime access to the course materials and free future updates and bonuses. (As I continue to update and add more valuable material to the course, you get it all for free)

Weight Loss Forever is a complete solution to weight loss and getting fit in the comfort and PRIVACY of your own home.

What you need:
· Small amount of space
· 1 or 2 pairs of light dumbbells. A pair of 1kg and a pair of 2kg are best.
· An exercise matt
· 20-30 minutes Two or Three days a week.
· A clean bill of health from your Doctor or General Practitioner to ensure you can start a new diet and exercise program.

No exercise experience necessary
No cooking or nutritional experience necessary

Go here for more information and to get a FREE 14 DAY PASS.

http://www.richard-clarke.co.uk/academy/

Date	Weight	Date	Weight